This book is available to you without charge with the belief that it offers you methods to improve the quality of your life and increase your chances of successfully fighting cancer. After you have read the book, please give it to another cancer patient. If you are unable to do this, please give it to a library or minister so that they may loan it to someone it can help.

We would appreciate hearing your feelings after you read this book. Drop us a note. We care about you!

Annette and Richard Bloch
The Cancer Hot Line
4400 Main Street
Kansas City, MO 64111
(816) 932-8453
(816) WE BUILD
(800) 433-0464

Annette and Richard Bloch

Fighting Cancer

A STEP-BY-STEP GUIDE
TO HELPING YOURSELF
FIGHT CANCER

Foreword by
Vincent T. DeVita, Jr., M.D.
Director of the National Cancer Institute
1980 – 1988

Published by
R.A. Bloch Cancer Foundation
4400 Main Street, Kansas City, Missouri 64111
816-932-8453
800-433-0464
www.blochcancer.org
A not-for-profit corporation

Dedication

This book is written for and dedicated to the people with cancer who want to do everything in their power to help themselves and their doctor so they will have the best chance of beating their disease.

Five days after I was told I had "terminal" lung cancer, another doctor told me he would cure me so I could work for cancer. I promised that if he did, I would. *Cancer...there's hope*, *Fighting Cancer* and *Guide for Cancer Supporters* are three of the many projects we are working on to fulfill that promise. We trust this book will provide you with the knowledge, hope, inspiration and desire to successfully fight your disease.

One woman wrote to us saying, "Last August 24, I had surgery for ovarian cancer. The doctor said the cancer had spread throughout the abdominal cavity and he saw no point in putting me through chemotherapy or radiation. He felt I should live whatever time I had left in peace and dignity. I refused to accept that and decided to read everything I could on my enemy. One of the first books I read was Richard Bloch's *Cancer...there's hope*. After reading this, I started practicing "imaging" and continued to read and practice attitudinal healing. When the doctor next saw me, he was so surprised at my appearance and progress, he decided to go ahead with chemotherapy. The cancer now seems to be localized in one mass that should be removable by surgery...I feel I owe a great deal to Mr. Bloch's books..."

We know everyone cannot beat cancer. If this book helps just one person overcome their problem, all our efforts will be worthwhile. Maybe that one person can be you.

Acknowledgements

Our sincerest gratitude to the wonderful doctors and other individuals without whose conscientious and dedicated time and assistance, this book would not have been possible:

Dr. Vincent T. DeVita, Jr., former director of the National Cancer Institute, and his very capable staff who assisted in reviewing this manuscript.

The outstanding medical oncologist, radiation oncologist, pathologist, diagnostic radiologist, surgeon and psychologist who, even though extremely busy, took their valuable time and meticulously went over this book, offering valuable comments and suggestions.

The well known and beloved minister who helped us examine the spiritual aspects of a life-threatening illness.

Our daughter, Linda Lyon, whose countless hours of editing and efforts in publishing made this book a reality.

And particularly to all those wonderful doctors who donated their efforts at the R.A. Bloch Cancer Management Center, from whose guidance and inspiration we were able to gain the knowledge to assemble this information.

Table of Contents

Foreword

This book is a product of Dick and Annette Bloch's own experience with cancer. The overriding message that cancer patients must utilize all available information to seek out the best possible care and do everything they can to maximize their chances for therapeutic success is a vital one. This is a strong personal statement about striving for life. It should motivate many cancer patients to obtain state-of-the-art treatment and to play an active part in increasing their own chances of being among the growing number of survivors.

Vincent T. DeVita, Jr., M.D.
Director, 1980 — 1988
National Cancer Institute

Introduction

Cancer is the most curable of all chronic diseases. Today, the goal is not merely to prolong life — the best that could be hoped for in the past — but to cure the patient of the disease.

Everyone cannot beat cancer. Some people are going to succumb to it. If you try to fight it, however, you have a chance of beating it.

This book is not written to entertain or lecture. It is written as concisely as possible by a layman in layman's language to help the individual who has cancer have the best possible chance of beating it.

Be positive! Start with the assumption that everything in this book applies to you. Don't be negative. Don't assume that anything may be fine for someone else but not for you. That particular constructive suggestion is specifically for you! Don't knock it until you have tried it. After you give it a fair trial, then and only then can you honestly say it isn't for you.

You are a unique person. You have been brought up with individual standards, practicing your own set of customs based on your beliefs from the experiences to which you were exposed. Not only is no one else identical to you, but they are not even similar to you. There will be many things in this book that you can readily identify with and completely understand. Other facets will seem contrary to your nature and beyond belief or comprehension. I urge you to remember that these are generally not only my personal opinions or beliefs; they are the recommendations of outstanding scientists, physicians and other professionals who deal with cancer patients regularly.

The only purpose in writing this book is to see that you have the best chance of beating cancer as easily as possible. We are not writing this book for money — we will never get one penny from it. We are not writing it for ego — we have had more than enough accolades even though we always like to see your letters. We are not writing this book to keep ourselves busy — there are more things we want to do than we have time for. We don't know you and probably will never meet you. We are writing this book for your benefit only!

Nothing is put in this book to fill space. You got it to help you fight cancer, not to keep you busy reading. It is not possible to emphasize enough how important every item expressed is to the assurance of recovery. Don't rationalize that one little item can be ignored without jeopardizing chances of recovery. That single factor that you have never heard of and probably doubt the validity of and may seem like a nuisance could be the key to recovery. Let me assure you that each thought has been originated by someone other than me. They have been discussed over and over by many people. They have been tried by numerous cancer patients before you and are believed to be a positive factor in recovery. Furthermore, nothing contained herein is believed to have any downside risk. Many other things could have been put in but might pose a potential risk for some people. It is believed that nothing in this book, if properly implemented, has any negative possibility.

We want to go on record cautioning you that these are only suggestions for you to try in a positive view. In all probability, every detail will not be constructive for each individual. Do not get guilty feelings if you try something and do not feel that it is helping you. Very rarely can anyone actually "feel" cancer leaving. It is very important, however, to try anything that is not harmful because it might help, but have no guilt feelings if it does not.

It is my personal opinion that the greatest cause of mortality from cancer is the individual equating death and cancer. When an individual is diagnosed with a malignancy, their first assumption is that it will eventually kill them, and they therefore do not muster all their resources to fight this vicious disease. Cancer is a word, not a sentence.

Often the physician who makes the initial diagnosis is a contributor to the problem. If he graduated medical school only 10 years ago, over half the cancers he was told were untreatable when he was in school are today curable to some degree. Furthermore, the physician has seen the suffering that went along with some of the primitive treatments in the past, and he cannot see putting his beloved patient through this. He recommends they go home and make themselves as comfortable as possible for the time they have to live.

I am not trying to say that everyone can beat cancer. Certainly some people are going to die from it, no matter what they do. I am saying, however, that if a person does not try, there is no way they can beat it. If they do try, they have a chance. And I believe it can do nothing but improve the quality of their life. To me, there was nothing worse than waiting to die with no hope. Whatever treatments I went through did not compare to the lack of hope I had the first 5 days after diagnosis. I was fighting to live rather than waiting to die.

It is believed that the average person gets cancer 6 times a year. Their immune system destroys the cancer cells, and they know nothing about it. Occasionally, something comes along to depress the immune system, which allows these malignant cells to get a foothold and multiply. When the immune system recovers, the cancer is already too well established and they have a detectable case of cancer. It is often discovered by a general doctor who tells the patient there is no hope, further depressing the immune system. The patient has complete confidence in this doctor who represents the entire medical system, so there is no purpose in getting a second opinion or going elsewhere. The patient is totally out of control at this point, compounding the problem.

There have been numerous studies documenting the effects of stress on the immune system, both with animals and individuals. It has been demonstrated that tumors grow faster in mice under stress. Mice have fared worse and died sooner when they were made to feel helpless. The incidence of cancer in individuals following a traumatic event such as the death of a spouse or child or retirement has been shown to increase dramatically. It has even been demonstrated that individuals with suicidal tendencies have a higher incidence of cancer, indicating that cancer could be a legal method of committing suicide.

Couple this with the fact that rarely is cancer ever diagnosed by an oncologist. Around 85% of all cancer patients do not use an oncologist as their primary physician. Cancer is an extremely complex array of over 100 different diseases with at least 6 common methods of treatment, any one of which could successfully treat some cancers, but generally they are given in combination. If it is not treated promptly, properly and thoroughly, there usually is no second chance. Progress in cancer treatments is being made at such a rapid pace that no single individual could conceivably know all the latest and best treatments for any single type of cancer, let alone all the different cancers.

It is for these reasons that I believe the greatest single mortality factor in cancer is the patient believing that death and cancer are synonymous. Promptly getting the patient to a multidisciplinary panel or to a board certified oncologist for a second opinion could do more to save lives than anything else. If they try, they have a chance. If they don't, they are as good as dead.

Cancer mortality has dropped for the first time in history! The age-adjusted cancer death rate declined from 1990 to 1995 3.1% from 135.0 per 100,000 population to 129.8, the lowest it has been in the preceding 25 years. Further, the decline is accelerating and continuing at about 2% per year.

This is attributed to earlier detection and improved treatments. We agree with this completely but believe they are failing to give credit to the psychological changes that have taken place in the same period. The public has been bombarded with stories of cancer successes. Individuals who were brought up to believe that a diagnosis of cancer was equivalent to impending death were suddenly aware that if they tried to fight, they had an excellent chance, better than 50%, of beating the disease. Further, that if they caught the disease earlier their chances of successful treatment were dramatically enhanced. And the treatments are not as bad as they had been touted because they have been improved.

One national figure in the cancer war stated, "It is likely that there will be a 25% decrease in the overall death rate from cancer, and possibly as much as 50% decrease, in the next 20 years." Progress is being made! There are two caveats in the data. First, the overall death rate, as compared to the age-adjusted death rate, continues to rise because the population is aging and cancer is a disease of old age. Physicians predict cancer will surpass heart disease as the nation's leading killer.

Second, while African Americans have shown substantial improvements, the overall death rate is still 33% higher in black men than in white men. We believe that this second factor is primarily due to black men believing they cannot get "as good" medical treatment and therefore not trying to beat it, or procrastinating. In every community we know of, state-of-the-art therapy is available to any cancer patient first, with payment due later. A great deal of publicity of this fact should substantially reduce the adverse mortality figures.

Understanding Cancer 1

There is no type of cancer from which some people have not recovered. The road to recovery generally is not very easy and requires real determination. Currently, the statistics show that over 60% of all serious cancers can be cured. The one item that you rationalize is a bother or does not apply to you can be the deciding factor that would tilt the scale in your favor or against you. You generally have one chance. Use every resource in your power.

Cancer is a unique disease. There are five factors that make it different from any other known illness. First, cancer cells grow geometrically without limitation. That means 2 becomes 4, then 8, 16, 32, 64, etc. If they grew 1, then 2, 3, 4, 5, we probably would never have heard of it. Because of this geometric growth, we must treat it promptly and properly or it can soon grow to a point where it may be untreatable. If we break our arm and it is not set properly, we can have it reset again whenever we want. It is not irreversible and terminal. (See chart on following page).

To further illustrate the way cancer grows, picture algae covering a lake. This algae doubles in area each day until, after one month's time, it completely covers the lake. When should it be noticed? When it covers one half of the lake? That is the day before the end of the month. When it only covers one fourth of the lake? That is two days before the end of the month. If you caught yours three or four or five days before the end of the month, you must feel very grateful!

The second unique factor is the property of cancer cells to spontaneously travel to distant sites. One million cancer cells are smaller than the head of a pin. One billion cancer cells are the size of a pea. This means that they have the ability to float freely through the blood stream or the lymph system. They could be in your stomach today

Growth and Detection of Cancer Cells

One million cancer cells are smaller than the head of a pin. One billion cancer cells are the size of a pea and weigh about the same as a paper clip. Below is a chart showing the geometric growth of cancer.

Number Of Cells

1	= The inception of cancer – one malignant cell growing uncontrollably.
10^1	= 10
10^2	= 100
10^3	= 1000
10^4	= 10,000 etc.
10^5	
10^6	
10^7	
10^8	
10^9	= The earliest that cancer will normally be detected by X-ray, scan, mammogram or feel.
10^{10}	
10^{11}	
10^{12}	
10^{13}	= The stage at which the patient is generally dead.

This chart is meant to emphasize two critical factors: the importance of early detection, and prompt treatment. Time is of the essence!

and in your head, your lungs or your toes tomorrow. If you break your arm, it cannot metastasize (spread) to your hip.

Third is that cancer is actually over 100 different diseases. There is no similarity between brain cancer and breast cancer other than the word cancer and the fact that they are both rapidly dividing cells. Different types of cancer should be treated by different types of medical specialists with totally different methods after being diagnosed through different means. Furthermore, the advances being made continuously in the many different types of treatments make it absolutely impossible for any one individual to know the very latest and best therapy for every type of cancer. In contrast, if you break your arm, many physicians would know the state-of-the-art way to set it.

Fourth is the unique fact that while many cancers can be treated successfully the first time, if they are not, often there is no second chance. For example, with my lung cancer, I had all the radiation my lung could take; so, if I had not been cured completely and had suffered a recurrence, I could not again have successfully had radiation therapy. I had my limit on Adriamycin, a particularly effective cancer drug but one which can do harm if given in excess of certain amounts, so it would not have been available to me if needed a second time. After you have one lung removed, there is no point in talking about surgery because you cannot live without both lungs. These are just examples in my case, but the same principles apply in many cases. This is why we not only preach prompt and proper treatment but also thorough treatment so you know you have the best chance of being through with it forever. If you break your arm a second time, generally it is not more critical than the first time.

Fifth and last is the major factor mental attitude plays in the recovery from cancer. Most oncologists agree that if a patient believes they will die from their cancer, they are right and cannot be saved. That is not to state that if they believe they will recover, they necessarily will, but at least they have a chance. If you break your arm, whether you think it will mend or not does not matter, it will generally heal in so many days.

Some people feel that because they don't have sufficient funds they won't receive the best treatments. In fact, these people are defeatists. They are making up their minds in advance that they are going to take the easy road out and give in to their disease. I have never seen the individual who, even though absolutely destitute, could not get the proper treatments if they applied themselves and really tried. There are resources in every major community. Remember, no one owes you anything. You have to work to get it like everything else in life. It can be done! An example of some of the resources that could be investigated are VA hospitals, state cancer hospitals, university hospitals or teaching institutions, and county or city hospitals. Treatment for patients participating in National Cancer Institute clinical research protocols at the Clinical Center of the National Institutes of Health is provided free of charge. Generally, a local, qualified physician can give you suggestions on where to look.

Some people have said I recovered because of my financial position and that I must have gotten preferential treatment. I would like to dispel this myth. First of all, I am unaware that cancer shows partiality because of financial or any other position. I believe rich or poor people have an equal chance of surviving. I also believe that tall or short people have a relatively equal chance as well as fat or thin or black or white people.

As to receiving preferential treatment, that was hardly the case. At home, where I was known and possibly could have gotten superior attention, I was told it was hopeless and to get my estate in order. If that is superior treatment, I don't need it. When I went 900 miles away to a mammoth institution where I was a number, I did receive superb service and attention, not because of who I was but because that is the way they do things. My doctor, before giving me any treatments, gave me his home telephone number. He said in the next two years of treatments I would want to contact him many times in the middle of the night or over the weekend. Of course, I could reach him during weekdays at the clinic. However, he did not want me to waste my energy during a sleepless night or weekend about anything that would be bothering me. He wanted me to apply all my energy to getting well. For that reason, he gave me his home telephone number and told me to call him any time anything bothered me. He did this for his other patients also, as should all good doctors.

This discussion of my doctor is only for the purpose of showing you where I got my support, ideas and knowledge and what you should look for and have a right to expect from your physician.

My doctor was the greatest! Not only did he cure me from cancer, but he taught me so much along the way. In the very first telephone conversation, he started, without my knowing it, by getting my undivided attention and ascertaining my dedication.

I was diagnosed on a Wednesday with "terminal" stage 3 squamous cell lung cancer. I talked with him Wednesday night long distance, and he wanted me to fly there Thursday so I could be examined and tested

Friday. The clinic is closed on Saturday and Sunday. Because I was terminal and might never have seen my home or office again, I wanted to have four days to get my estate in order at the expense of one day of testing. I wanted to fly down Sunday to be examined and tested on Monday, one working day later. My doctor said if I did not fly down on Thursday, he would not treat me.

At the time, I may have thought he was being inconsiderate. Since then, that one little remark has taught me many things. First of all, cancer is never as treatable as it is right now! At some time in the future, it is probably not treatable. Whether that time is tomorrow, next week or next month depends on the individual case. This afternoon or first thing tomorrow morning is the best time to start trying to beat it.

Possibly even more important than that, I soon came to realize he wanted to be certain that recovering from cancer had my full attention. He wanted to be certain that I would make the commitment to do whatever was necessary to get well. There is no doubt that generally it is a long, hard road with plenty of obstructions and detours. He wanted to be sure that I wasn't going to say, "OK, Doc. I'll do anything you tell me to do as long as it is convenient with me." He wanted to know that getting well came first before anything and everything else in my life.

And possibly the most important thing I learned from those few words was a third factor. He wanted to know that I had the dedication and drive to do what would be required to be victorious over cancer. That day may not have been critical. But that day represented just one of the many negative options that would lie in the path of my recovery that I would have to forgo if I were going to succeed. He knew my chances of recovery were much greater if I had a truly strong, burning desire to live. This was his way of testing me. This was his way of proving it. If I would give up four days I wanted so desperately to give him his one day he asked for, my dedication to success was guaranteed.

The biggest and the hardest single thing that you will be required to do in the entire battle is to make up your mind to really fight it. You must, on your own, make the commitment that you will do everything in your power to fight your disease. No exceptions. Nothing halfway. Nothing for the sake of ease or convenience. Everything! Nothing short of it. When you have done this, you have accomplished the most difficult thing you will have to accomplish throughout your entire treatment. This applies no matter how serious or how minor you are led to believe your cancer is.

If it is minor, great. Your commitment should not be difficult to abide by. If you are told you are going to die in 3 months or 3 years or whatever, then your commitment is that much more vital. There are a lot of "terminal" people alive, healthy and cancer free. There is no type of cancer from which some people have not been cured. There is no cancer for which there is no treatment.

To give up requires no commitment. You can stay in the comfort of your own lifestyle. Fighting means a complete change of lifestyle, absolutely leaving your comfort zone. There will be doctors doing things you might not like. There will be lots of work for you to do. There might even be some pain and suffering, and certainly lots of new and unexpected experiences. You must decide that the end is worth the means because you are the only one who can do it. No one else can do it for you. There is no half way. It's all the way. But when it is all said and done, no matter what the results are, I've never met anyone who felt it was not the best way. Go for it with no second thoughts or regrets.

Remember, once you have made the commitment, everything else is relatively easy. There will be pleasant experiences. There will be unpleasant experiences. But I can promise you it is not as difficult as making the decision to make the commitment.

Fighting cancer is not a simple matter of thinking positively, wishing it away and saying, "Hey doc, cure me." It is a matter of knowledge. It is a matter of educating yourself about every detail and mustering all your resources. Use every drop of energy in an organized fashion to constructively concentrate on getting rid of cancer. Most cancers can be successfully treated, but generally you have only one chance. If you miss that first chance, if you don't do everything in your power, often there is no second chance. This is why no cancer patient can afford the luxury of looking back and saying, "I wish I would have..." Never look back. Concentrate on this moment forward and do everything in your power. There is no downside risk. Now you may have a chance.

The Act of Deciding to Fight Cancer

Until you commit yourself, there is hesitancy, the chance to draw back, ineffectiveness. Once you commit yourself to do absolutely everything in your power to fight cancer, all sorts of positive things occur. The mere act of reaching a decision causes unforeseen incidents, meetings and assistance that could not have been anticipated. Goethe stated, "Whatever you can do or dream you can, begin it. Boldness has genius, power and magic in it." *You* make it happen.

When I talk to a cancer patient who is still smoking (including but not limited to lung or throat cancer), the answer as to why that person continues to smoke is obvious without asking the question. Way down deep this person knows that smoking is bad for them.

No one has to explain. No one has to plead with them to give it up. What this person is saying–no, what this person is screaming to me is that they only want to live as long as it is easy and convenient for them. They are not willing to do anything and everything to help their doctor cure them. They know they must do everything in their power if they want to have a chance of getting well. By continuing to smoke, they are saying that they are not willing to do everything in their power to be cured, and therefore their chances are dramatically reduced. Maybe that is their privilege, but they should not ask others to do everything possible if they are not willing to help themselves.

I talked with a 42 year old lady paralyzed from the waist down with cancer from an undetermined origin. She had been told she would never walk again. Asked if she smoked, she replied that she knew it was bad for her and had been meaning to give it up long before she got cancer. As soon as she could get up on crutches and walk, she was going to go to a hypnotist to quit. This told me that if she didn't change her attitude, she would defeat herself. She obviously loved smoking and was dependent on it. She had promised to quit as soon as she could walk. She might have subconsciously procrastinated in her attempt to walk in order to delay as long as possible her quitting smoking.

Annette called my doctor out of the hospital room one morning to ask him a question about me. He marched her right back and gave her quite a tongue lashing in front of me. He told her never to ask him a question about me except in front of my face. There could be no secrets from a cancer patient if there was any hope that patient could get well. That single event probably did more constructive good for my mental attitude than any other factor. Just to realize that I was told everything honestly about my condition removed all doubts.

One day in the clinic we asked my doctor if a friend of ours, who he was treating, would make it. His reply startled us. He said we could talk to him and look into his eyes and know as well as he did whether this person would recover. We tried it. This person's posture was terribly bent over; his walk was a shuffle like someone 40 years older; his yellowish, sagging skin and head and face without a hair made him look like death warmed over; yet, the accent and genuine determination in his voice and glint in his eyes made us believe he was going to make it. And this was in spite of the fact that 85% of his liver had been replaced by cancer. And you know what! For several months thereafter, we got reports on how his tumor shrank and his liver regenerated itself. Truly a miracle.

The opposite had also been true. I talked with two volunteers at the Cancer Hot Line training program. Both of these women had experienced breast cancer. They had been treated by fine oncologists and had been told they were cured. One of them felt very depressed whenever she talked to anyone with cancer, and the other could not stand to even mention cancer. I came home and told my wife that I did not believe either of these people were through with their cancer in spite of what they had been told by their physicians. Today, one of those two is gallantly fighting against recurrent breast cancer and the other has passed away.

I wish there were an easy way to specifically list the points to take into account to render an accurate psychological prognosis. As each case of cancer is as unique as a fingerprint, so is each person's desire and determination. To camouflage it as a positive attitude is oversimplification.

In a visit to Pittsburgh for a press conference on the opening of a new Cancer Hot Line, I was picked up at the airport by a woman with an extremely positive attitude. She knew she was going to make it. She was in her fourth recurrence of breast cancer. She had the finest oncologist, in her words, in Allegheny County. I asked what his prognosis was. She told me she had never asked him because she did not want to hear what he would say. She knew she would beat it! What did this tell me? She had a qualified oncologist in whom she had complete confidence. She was afraid to ask him about her future, believing he doubted she could ever recover. Therefore, down deep, she believed she would not make it. Sure enough, a few months later she passed away.

Failure to become intimately involved with all the details of your cancer is like closing your eyes after falling into quicksand. For the moment maybe, your ignorance will give you a false sense of security. However, to have a chance of escaping, you must muster all your resources and use and exhaust every option open to you.

Hamilton Jordan, White House Chief of Staff under President Jimmy Carter, upon being diagnosed with cancer at the age of 41, stated, "One of my closest friends is a doctor, and he came to see me one day and said, 'You're going to have to manage your own damn medical care.' That shocked me. It put a sense of burden and responsibility on me that I wasn't sure I could exercise properly. But as I saw things unfold, I saw he was right. Although it was tempting to stay at (the hospital) and be among all my friends, and the (hospital) doctors thought they could do as good a job as anybody, I realized there were many choices to be made, and I had to make them for myself."

One of the major problems is that the initial diagnosis, while traumatic and beyond comprehension, is often relatively innocuous. It is often discovered through a routine physical examination, surgery for another situation or a question about some minor symptom. Some people feel that maybe it isn't as bad as it is cracked up to be and maybe, if they do nothing, it will just fade away. These individuals are looking in exactly the wrong direction. They should be grateful that their cancer was discovered at such an early stage and then promptly do everything in their power to successfully treat it.

The initial diagnosis of cancer makes many feel they have totally lost control. It is vital to get some part of this control back. The patient and the entire family faces a multitude of decisions. It is helpful to the patient and the family if the strategy is openly discussed and defined so that all members understand it. Also, the more information you have, the more power you can have to deal with the situation. By gaining knowledge, you can get back some of your control.

This is your life, and you are entitled to make your own decisions, but only if you have adequate information to make good decisions. These are all human judgments because no one has a God-given power to make them. Information will help you feel some personal control and security during treatment. The peace of mind gained by knowledge is an important factor in healing.

There are many sources for this information. Make a list of what you would like to know to ask your doctor the next time you talk to him. He is usually more than willing to explain anything you want to know. Look up your disease and the treatments in the public library or on your computer. I recommed OncoLink, NCI or www.blochcancer.org. Call 1-800-4-CANCER (U.S. Government Cancer Information Service), a Cancer Hot Line, the American Cancer Society, the Leukemia Society or other appropriate support groups. They generally have a great deal of information available that they will be happy to send to you and answer your questions. It often proves helpful to talk to someone who has had the same problem. This can be arranged through your doctor or a support group.

At a meeting of the psychiatrists and psychologists who donated their services at the R.A. Bloch Cancer Management Center, a discussion was had of the priority of the various goals they try to accomplish. It was determined that one objective stood out above all others: that of ascertaining the patient's support mechanism. Whether it be family, friends, neighbors, paid people such as a companion, nurse or doctor, the most important single controllable factor in your recovery is to establish a good support organization.

Stress and depression are integral parts of this disease. The sooner we realize that, the better and easier they are to cope with. We must have outlets to vent our emotions and support us in times of need. No matter how strong we each think we are, without a good support mechanism we will crumble.

At the initial trauma of being diagnosed, a person will mistakenly feel that they do not want to burden their loved ones with the depressing aspects of the disease. They will feel that they do not want to bore or inflict their discomfort on their friends or neighbors. Nothing could be further from reality. Your family who love you want to show their love by sharing your feelings with you. Your friends want to express their support by understanding your problems and trying to help you with them. You are not imposing on them by opening up. You are allowing them to do what they deeply and sincerely want to do by sharing your emotions and feelings with them. If you shut them out of your life, you are not doing them or yourself any favor. It may be hard to believe at first, but it makes no difference how old or how young they are or how strong or how infirm they are, everyone you know wants honestly to help you and is capable in some degree to help you. You are hurting them by saying you don't want them to. Allow them in. Make them feel wanted. Let them share and do their thing. It is one of those situations where everyone wins. Everyone is better off.

In Neil Simon's *Brighton Beach Memoirs*, Eugene, 14, mentions Aunt Blanche, "You see, her husband, Uncle Dan, died six years ago from...this thing. They never say the word. They always whisper it. It was (he whispers) cancer! I think they are afraid if they said it out loud, God would say, 'I heard that! You said the dread disease. Just for that, I smite you down with it.' There are some things that grown-ups just won't discuss." For many cancer patients, the reticence and awkwardness of acquaintances is an additional burden.

When talking about your problem with anyone, always include a statement to the effect, "With the help of my wonderful doctors, family and friends, we are going to do everything in our power to beat this disease." It would not be wrong to state when appropriate, "Even though the statistics for my problem are (not) terrible, I am not a statistic. I am going to do everything possible to be one of those who survive this."

Make a written list of your support mechanism. In addition to family, friends, neighbors, companions, office co-workers, tradespeople, and professionals, don't forget to include volunteers and organized support groups. Many are organized for the prime purpose of helping you. Help them by allowing them to help you. On your list, next to the name of each member of your support team, write a date on which you will contact them if you have not heard from them. When you make contact, cross this date off and put the next date to contact down. By doing this, you will be helping them and yourself.

Rabbi Hirshel Jaffe, in his book *Why Me, Why Anyone* states, "I feel more in command of things. Strangely, somehow I feel more alive. By facing death I am learning how to live. I've learned you shouldn't feel cursed if you have a disease with a foul name. Don't think of yourself as worthless because you've been stricken. Tell the people you love how you feel about them while you still have the chance. Be kind to yourself. We should be thankful for each day granted to us and treat it joyously. Every moment is special to me."

Cancer is often an eye-opener, teaching us that life is too short to postpone what we really want. It starts us thinking about how much we really enjoy life. In that respect, it can really be a positive experience because those who have cancer can use it in positive ways, to grow and to change their ways for the better and to profoundly affect the lives of loved ones around them in deeply positive ways.

Initial Approach 2

According to Dr. Shlomo Breznitz, a visiting Israeli psychologist at the National Institute of Mental Health, there are four styles of response to the initial diagnosis of cancer. The first is hope. Hoping is an active process in which one imagines a positive future based on a realistic assessment of the present. Hope does not blot out the bad. Instead, it emphasizes the positive.

The second style, hope plus denial, is an illusion. People who "hope for the best" may fall apart when faced with bad news.

Third, total denial, is when the person blocks out the problem entirely. Denial is a psychological sign showing the person is unwilling to confront reality.

Giving up, the fourth style, means neither hoping nor denying and has the worst prognosis.

Norman Cousins, in his book entitled *Human Options*, states, "One's confidence or lack of it, in the prospects of recovery from serious illness affects the chemistry of the body. The belief system converts hope, robust expectations, and the will to live into plus factors in any contest of forces involving disease. The belief system is not just a state of mind. It is a prime physiological reality. It is the application of options to the maintenance of health and the fight against disease. It is the master switch that gets the most out of whatever is possible. The greatest force in the human body is the natural drive of the body to heal itself–but that force is not independent of the belief system, which can translate expectations into physiological change. Nothing is more wondrous about the fifteen billion neurons in the human brain than their ability to convert thoughts, hopes, ideas, and attitudes into chemical substances. Everything begins, therefore, with belief. What we believe is the most powerful option of all."

Norman Cousins indicates that he was cured from an extremely serious illness primarily by exposing himself to humor and laughing. Somehow, laughter can stir up positive hormones in the body. Expose yourself to humor and things that make you laugh whenever possible. Some hospitals have put laughing rooms in the oncology departments, so there must be something to this. Don't pass it up as one of the many ways to help yourself. Appreciate the philosophy of laughter!

The Jonsson Comprehensive Cancer Center at UCLA tested strolling musicians, from a large surgical floor all the way to pediatrics, where live music calmed crying babies hooked to machines. Children with leukemia, each in an isolation room with only a small window to the hall, stood on step stools to see and hear the music. Three other visual arts programs are flourishing there, including art exhibits by fine artists who have experienced cancer. Their hope is that these concepts will be available in all cancer centers.

Keep yourself mentally and physically active during the term of your recuperation.

Take courses, attend study groups, continue to work if possible, read books, participate in church or outreach groups or anything you would enjoy doing. Follow through and do these things even though sometimes you have to push yourself to do them.

It is important that you exercise regularly. Talk to your doctor about this. Whether this exercise is merely a simple isometric like tensing and relaxing different muscles of your body or walking or whatever you are able to do, the important thing is to do something regularly.

On the other hand, be selfish. Don't overdo. Give in to yourself when you are tired or not feeling well. Recognize in advance that your recuperation will not always be a smooth easy road. It will have its ups and downs. Some days will be worse than others. Give in to yourself on those days. But remember that whenever you can, push yourself to do some kind of activity.

Don't mistake the side effects of the treatments for the symptoms of the disease. Many treatments can make you tired, weak or upset your stomach. This is absolutely normal and expected and could even indicate that the treatments are doing their job rather than the disease is getting worse.

A woman called and said she had just been diagnosed as having cancer and was afraid of dying. That is a very normal reaction and certainly nothing to be ashamed of. I think all of us probably felt exactly the same way, but most of us wouldn't admit it. To feel any other way would be abnormal. It is a good thing to get this out in the open, because once we can state a problem, we can often find a solution.

There are two aspects to face in that woman's statement in order to resolve it. First is that death and cancer are anything but synonymous. Most cancers can be successfully treated. The five year survival reported in 1982 was 46%, excluding skin and certain cervical cancers that are supposedly 100% curable. The figure for 1984 was 49% which is the relative survival for the period 1976-1981 because of the time delay in collecting the data. The 2002 figure was 62%. Furthermore, it is my personal opinion that if every patient had been treated promptly, properly and thoroughly by qualified physicians and had done everything else possible to help themselves, the figure would have been substantially higher.

Second is the aspect of being afraid to die, an absolutely normal and rational thought but one which deserves reconsideration at this stage of the game. The greatest damage will be done if we don't face it. The more an individual tries to avoid fear, the greater that fear will grow. Denying fear is costly in terms of personal energy. Suppressed fear will not dissipate but will continue to sap a person's energy. It is particularly harmful to a patient who needs all his resources to combat his disease. It will not help to try to suppress the fear. Get it out in the open so that it can be relieved.

Fear is an absolutely normal response to a life-threatening disease. The only danger to fear is when we deny it. Once fear is expressed and admitted, an excellent antidote can be knowledge.

After you have faced up to the fact that you have a life-threatening disease from which you might die, concentrate all your thoughts on living and fighting cancer.

We are all human beings. One hundred years from now we will all be dead. This was a fact when we were born, and we have always known it. The only question is "when." In my opinion, the quality of life is better for one who is fighting to live than one who is waiting to die. There is no possible way that searching for the state-of-the-art therapy and taking it could shorten your life one minute, and maybe it could lengthen it.

We cannot overcome our fear until we admit it. After we finally face up to our fear, there are ways to overcome it and learn to exist with it. Coming to terms with cancer means that denial must give way to free, healthy expressions of grief and fear. Moving from denial to realizing fear and anger can bring positive responses in many ways. The belief that our life has had meaning can lessen the fear of dying. The quality of our daily life affects our ability to handle fear. Being active and doing things you like gives less time to brood about your condition which, in itself, enhances your fear by allowing you to think about negative factors. Just the simple act of making a decision can give you a sense of moving forward and gaining purpose, of being in control.

From time to time, depression and negative thoughts will cross your mind. If they didn't, you would not be normal. Anger, impatience and selfishness are absolutely normal and could even be considered positive reactions. The one thing you must avoid is continued depression. The mere diagnosis of cancer causes depression. Many cancer treatments are depressing. Depression decreases the function of your immune system. Your immune system fights cancer. It is important that when you do find yourself depressed, you shake this feeling. Do this by talking about your depression to your family or friends. Change your thoughts from depressing subjects to positive, pleasant subjects. Channel the energy you would waste in depression into more positive thoughts. Concentrate all available energy into fighting your cancer.

There is an old saying, "Worry is like a rocking chair. It keeps you busy but gets you nowhere." Make up your mind that you have lots of things to do and lots of places to go. Whenever you feel yourself getting worried or depressed, try to change the direction of your thoughts and think about a forthcoming event. Plan things to do when you are with a particular relative or friend. Concentrate on your pleasant surroundings or try to recall some of the enjoyable situations you recently experienced or one of the many wonderful blessings with which you have been endowed. In other words, keep looking at the donut and not at the hole. Continuously plan new projects and goals that are realistic and attainable.

Common sense does not always give the best results, regardless of our intentions. We need to know how to help ourselves. If we allow ourselves to feel like a victim, we feel we have no control over our situation. We can't control everything in our lives, but we can learn to become an active participant and have a strong influence on what happens to us. Helplessness increases fear, anxiety and depression and can even cause a person to lose their will to live.

We are conditioned to believe that sick people are victims. With a long-term chronic illness, it is important to correct this attitude. Victims are often resentful toward their doctor, their family and everything else. While it is certainly understandable that anyone with cancer will feel like a victim at times, we must get back in control of ourselves so that we will not feel helpless, hopeless, and depressed.

Not only the disease but the side effects of the treatments can cause fatigue and emotional stress that can lead to depression. Long-term depression can be harmful to the cancer patient because it builds. We may not even be aware of it because we are taught it is not right, we are frightened of being depressed or we are worried about what others might think. When we deny it to the point that we are not aware of it, it is most critical because it will continue to sap our emotional and physical strength until resolved.

Acknowledging the existence of depression will not make it get worse. Admitting that we are depressed can give us the strength to overcome it. That in itself can give us hope and a better quality of life.

The day after I was diagnosed and told to get my estate in order, I was at my desk prior to going to Houston. I wrote a long letter to my family basically describing my feelings and emotions. While I didn't want to die and while I felt I was just beginning to reap the rewards for which I had worked 52 years, I had no regrets. I believe writing this letter helped me lessen my fear of dying. I gave it to one of my daughters to hold and open only in the event of my death. After I recovered from surgery some months later and felt confident that I was on the road to recovery, I got the letter back from her and put it with my will. Maybe something like this could help you. Often, when you talk something out or write about something that bothers you, it will stop troubling you.

An M.D. Anderson trained pediatric oncologist stated that he always discusses death and dying with each patient and their family because it is always a possibility in some types of cancer. He wanted to bring it out to avoid the patient's often unspoken fear of it. However, he treated each patient, regardless of their prognosis, as if they were going to live.

After he discusses the possibility of dying, his theory is to put all energy and thought into working toward living. When asked about certain professionals' belief that a person must prepare himself to die, his answer was, "That is nonsense." He has seen patients, who recovered after they were supposedly given no chance of recovery, have a difficult time adjusting to living. He has never seen a patient have a problem adjusting to death. It may have been a blunt way of putting it, but think about that statement for a minute. It is an undebatable truism.

He said that "terminal" is a place where you catch a bus and does not usually apply to a disease. Furthermore, he is not treating people who are dying. He is treating patients who are trying to live. Another outstanding cancer researcher, Dr. Jimmie Holland, states, "People ... are fighters and they want to fight to the end. They don't want to get the feeling that they have been given up. They want to be a part of the cutting edge of the fight against cancer."

Cancer is a serious disease, or really an assortment of over 100 different diseases. There are often many options in treatments. Such rapid progress is being made that no single physician is capable of knowing the very latest and best treatments for every type of cancer. Dr. Vincent T. DeVita, Jr., former director of the National Cancer Institute, stated that anyone with a life-threatening disease should seek a qualified second opinion. He says, "The worst thing a physician can do is to declare a patient 'incurable.' In that context, where the patient has confidence in his doctor, the doctor will always be needlessly correct."

Furthermore, he says, "I've been taking care of cancer patients for a long time. I have never taken care of a doctor who didn't get a second opinion. I've never taken care of a doctor who didn't have his microscopic slides read twice, by more than one pathologist, to make sure that he had cancer, knowing already that he had gotten into a pretty good system. And I think there is a message in that.

"One caution when seeking a second opinion is to be certain you truly receive an independent second opinion and not a second first opinion. Do not allow your doctor to refer you to his professor who taught him the way to do it, to his golfing buddy or to his co-worker in the same office. Be certain to look for a qualified, competent physician, separately trained and working in a different institution. Only in this way can you avoid getting a second first opinion."

In an annual review meeting of the National Cancer Institute, he stated that only 40% of the women in Los Angeles with breast cancer who should be getting adjuvant chemotherapy are receiving it. Sixty percent are not. Sixty percent of the women who have been described in every conservative study as needing treatment are not receiving it. And that is in a geographic area where supposedly superior attention is provided. When asking Dr. Bernard Fisher about this, he said that if you were to include people getting improper treatments, he would assume the figure nationally is much higher than 60%. This dramatically demonstrates the need for a qualified, independent second opinion.

As to whether you should go to a major cancer center for treatment, Dr. DeVita states, "Experience is what really counts in this whole business...If you had cancer, wouldn't you rather go to someone who had a lot of experience managing that cancer?" If your local doctor has had the experience of successfully treating your type of cancer, and a qualified, independent second opinion agrees with his recommended action, there should be no reason to go away from your community.

Dr. DeVita says patients have "got to be able to go to their doctors and ask a very simple question: 'Doctor, do you take care of this kind of cancer often?' If he says, 'Well, I treat two or three patients a year,' I think you should say, 'Could you find me somebody with experience?' Then telephone Cancer Information Service, and we can help you find the people with experience...That's the real crux of the situation ...The answer for anybody who has cancer is to go find the people who have experience. That is not always in a big cancer center. For example, our cancer center in Bethesda is one of the finest in the world. We study certain kinds of cancers, but there are certain kinds of cancers that we don't study at all. So for the ones that we don't study at all, we're not a good place to go.

"We're large, but if you had some kinds of cancer, we'd be small in terms of experience. Almost every center in the country that I know of is that way, with only a couple of exceptions...But most of the cancer centers have a personality because of the researchers they have attracted. They see a lot of one kind of cancer and not much of another kind; they study certain kinds. It's very hard for the public to identify the centers that have great expertise in one area and not in another.

"Patients are so shy about going to their doctor and saying, 'You know, doctor, you just told me I have cancer, and you said my chances are 50/50.' They are facing a 50% chance of losing their lives and they're shy about saying, 'I want to go to somebody who has experience.' And the doctor says, 'I don't have any experience but...' They seem to be shy about saying, 'Well, I'd rather go to somebody with experience.' Doctors intimidate people...Experience is what counts."

It is my personal opinion that most doctors do not intimidate patients. They are usually caring and compassionate. They put the patient's interest first and will voluntarily suggest a second opinion. However, you are not interested in most doctors. The only thing that matters to you is your doctor! If he is not caring and compassionate, if you do not relate well or feel comfortable with him or if he in any way discourages a second opinion, I would strongly suggest finding another doctor who meets these requirements.

A boy in North Carolina had Burkitt's lymphoma. The father telephoned Dr. Burkitt in London. He advised them there were two centers in America where there are leading experts in treating this: the National Cancer Institute in Washington and M.D. Anderson in Houston. "You couldn't go anywhere better in the world than these two places. I am not the right person to treat the boy. I would be 20 years behind these experts in treatment knowledge."

The National Cancer Institute, with the cooperation of 150 cancer centers in the United States and more than 22 foreign countries, has spent tremendous resources to place every known treatment for each kind of cancer on a computer. Furthermore, this is updated for each kind of cancer every month after being reviewed by 72 physicians and scientists. This information, called PDQ, is available free through your personal computer or by telephone. It is written in common, understandable English. It not only shows the state-of-the-art therapy for each kind of cancer along with statistics, but all other options including where successful experimental therapy is being done and who to talk to. It is also available to any physician, any patient or anyone else absolutely free by calling 1-800-4-CANCER and specifically requesting PDQ for the specific type and stage of cancer including all current open protocols.

In a government publication entitled *National Cancer Program*, it states, "If physicians avail themselves of the opportunity now offered by PDQ, the NCI estimates that national survival rates would rise by at least 10 percent, or more than 50,000 lives saved per year."

One morning a cancer patient, her husband and daughter came into my office. She was worried because she was to get no treatment other than radiation therapy. I was confident her fears were psychological. Her primary doctor was a superb medical oncologist. I had heard her type of cancer discussed numerous times at the Cancer Management Center, and radiation was the only treatment recommended.

Realizing that most people feel better when they read the recommendation themselves from an authoritative source, I turned to my trusty computer immediately behind my desk. In two minutes, I had a print-out of the current PDQ state-of-the-art treatment for her type of cancer. I read with her that the recommendation for her stage of cancer was solely radiation with excellent expected results. The only exception was when the initial spread was to a specific area of the body, which hers was, when the chance of a fatal recurrence without chemotherapy was nearly universal. We agreed that for the benefit of the doctor's pride, she would forget she was at my office. She would call her doctor and insist he get PDQ so he could "discover" this information on his own. One life was probably saved because a woman refused to wait and look back and say, "I wish I would have..."

Every cancer patient who is interested in recovering, and we must assume that since you are reading this book, you are interested in recovering, should insist that their doctor get a printout of the current PDQ as it pertains to their disease, and the patient should read it. Understand all your options. Know what your time frames are. Look into your future. Educate yourself in every possible way. Knowledge is power. It can help you help yourself fight cancer. Uncertainty and doubt stimulate stress which in turn depresses your immune system. Get PDQ, digest the information and know you are proceeding in the right direction and doing everything possible to help yourself.

Progress in the treatment of cancer is moving so rapidly that the state-of-the-art statements in PDQ were modified on an average of 15 per month during one 18 month period.

A publication of the National Institutes of Health entitled *Cancer Control Objectives for the Nation 1985-2000*, states, "The application of the state-of-the-art treatment is complex. At all levels of the health service delivery system from the primary care physician who has initial contact with the patient to specialists directing the cancer treatment physician knowledge is not yet optimal. That knowledge should include an appreciation for state-of-the-art treatment information and an interest in ensuring early multidisciplinary decision making...For about 70% of cancers, optimal therapy derives from multidisciplinary discussions. The relative rarity of some of the most responsive tumors means that proficient treatment can be maintained only at some major cancer centers... Malpractice considerations may result in physicians selecting 'safe' therapy, which neither offers significant risk nor the chance of cure...A major determinant of outcome for most newly diagnosed cancer patients with curable disease hinges on early multidisciplinary treatment planning and the availability of expertise and resources to carry out such a treatment plan." This is repeated again in Monograph No. 2 published by the National Cancer Institute.

Most cancers can be successfully treated if they are treated promptly, properly and thoroughly. As has been pointed out, you generally have only one chance to cure cancer. If it is not done right the first time, often there is no second chance. For this reason, I recommend a second opinion in every case of cancer, whatever the prognosis. If it is good, you want to be certain it is correct and if it is not, then you want other cancer doctors' opinions so you will know what can be done. The most important physician in the treatment of cancer is the pathologist. The necessity of treating the correct type of cancer from the start is paramount. Pathology is as important to the successful construction of a proper treatment as a solid foundation is to a large building. Without an accurate diagnosis, the others are left helpless.

One woman, four months pregnant, was told from a Pap smear that she had cervical cancer. Her doctor recommended an abortion and hysterectomy immediately. The pathologist discovered it was cervical cancer "in situ" which would not turn into cancer before 3 to 30 years from then. She was advised to have the baby without concern, after which the treatment for an absolute cure was simple.

A man had a malignant polyp removed from his colon. He was told they got it all out, that it was an indolent type of cancer, and he should do nothing but be watched. A pathologist found that it was a highly invasive type of cell and had probably not entirely been removed because it went to the edges of the tissue which was taken. Prompt surgery was recommended to remove a few inches of his colon, which meant cure if it had not penetrated through the wall, and additional treatments if it had.

A woman was sent back from a major cancer center with an active tumor of unknown origin and told to make herself as comfortable as possible. Nothing could be done. The pathologist stated that this cell generally came from one of two sources–the lung or the thyroid. They had wonderful X-rays and scans of the lung which were absolutely clear. He asked if she ever had cancer of the thyroid. She replied, "Of course not. But I did have a growth removed from my thyroid two years ago that was benign." They went back and got the tissues from that surgery which were found malignant and were able to recommend successful treatments.

A 74-year-old gentleman was told he had cancer of the pancreas with no hope. A pathologist found it was not malignant! To be certain, he, on his own, got opinions from three other pathologists who agreed. Not to leave any stone unturned, they sent the slides to the Armed Forces Institute of Pathology in Washington.

Most people never even get to meet their pathologist. In many cases, he can be the most critical doctor because if his conclusion is inaccurate, all the other doctors involved will be working on the wrong premise.

Now that you have the proper pathology, it is vital to receive the optimal treatments. In most types of cancer there are several options based not only on the individual's specific case, but on the patient's desires and lifestyle. What could be best for one patient might not be desirable for another. After being fully informed of all of their options, the patient should make the proper decision. The problem being presented here is how to become fully informed.

Many physicians are inclined to favor their own specialty for many reasons while other specialities could be more curative, less invasive, less debilitating or cause fewer side effects. Some physicians tend to favor what they are most familiar with and know the best. They have faith in what they can do. That is why they went into this field.

However, circumstances may have changed. New therapies may have been developed. Other specialists may have knowledge about which they are unaware. For a very few, it could even be a desire to produce revenue.

As previously stated, most cancers can be successfully treated, but you generally have only one chance. You want to be sure to embark on the proper therapy the first time. You want to get honest opinions from specialists in each discipline that could apply to your type of cancer. The best way to insure honest, forthright information is to have all the specialists who could have a therapy applicable to your particular type of cancer assembled simultaneously while each explains to you what they would recommend. This is what is known as a true multi-disciplinary second opinion.

The purpose of having the appropriate physicians together in front of you is many fold. First, it will keep you from getting the wrong interpretation from a physician's statement. Most important, you can hear all the options available substantiated with the success rates rather than hearing one specialist's biased opinion. Also, knowing all your options and making an informed decision will not only give you peace of mind, but will enhance your confidence in the treatments and augment your chance of success.

We are presently soliciting various institutions around the United States to make this type of multidisciplinary second opinion available to newly diagnosed cancer patients. Check with your physician or a major institution near you to see if it is available in your vicinity. If you cannot locate one, call the Cancer Information Service at 1-800-4-CANCER or the Bloch Cancer Hot Line at 800-433-0464.

While it is easier to rely on the first opinion you get, particularly if it is a favorable prognosis, please don't bet your life on it. A second opinion is vital, and if there is more than one option possible, it should be received directly and simultaneously from each specialist involved. The quality of life and peace of mind you derive from a qualified second opinion will prove well worthwhile.

Code of Practice at the
R.A. Bloch Cancer
Management Center

To Achieve Excellence
Attempt Perfection
Less is Unacceptable

Medical Treatments 3

There are two schools of thought on patient education. One is for the patient not to know, to care or to worry. Let the doctor or other health professional treat and cure you. The other is to explain every aspect of the disease and treatment so the patient can understand and become an active participant, not a recipient. Today, oncologists (doctors specially trained to treat cancer) are taught the latter method. It is believed the greatest resource to cure a patient is within the patient.

There is an old tale with a great moral called the "wheelbarrow story." An individual carted scrap metal from machines in a plant to the junk pile hour after hour, day after day. The turnover in this position had been high, and the current employee was very slow and lethargic. The plant manager came to him one day and explained the entire process of producing their product and what an important place this individual had in continuously moving the scrap from the machine to the junk pile. He was an integral and vital cog in the entire operation. From that moment on, he did an outstanding job.

I believe the same thing applies in the recovery from cancer. If we can understand the part that we are able to perform, we can help ourselves do an outstanding job in the successful treatment of our disease. It is for that reason that the following information on medical treatment is presented. It is so that you can understand what your options are, what your doctor is recommending, why it is being recommended, what it is intended to do and how it is supposed to do it. With this information, it is hoped that your mind and your body will help the treatments do their intended job.

This book could not serve you well without some discussion of alternative therapies. Even though you have cancer, you still have a good mind, and you are able to think and rationalize. You have gone through a traumatic experience being diagnosed with cancer, but that doesn't mean you have to rush into everything with blind faith and believe everything anyone says or everything you read. Use the common sense God gave you without trying to take the easy road out.

There are three types of treatments that you must consider in treating cancer. First are orthodox medical treatments (such as surgery, chemotherapy, and the other treatments described later in this chapter) of which I am completely in favor when prescribed by a qualified physician and concurred with by an independent qualified second opinion. Orthodox medical treatments always come first and foremost in treating cancer.

Second are termed supplemental (such as prayer, relaxation, imagery and diet), which means methods of treatment that are used in addition to orthodox medical treatments. I am completely in favor of any and all supplemental forms of treatment as long as your physician says they will not specifically harm you or interfere with whatever medical treatments you are taking.

Third are alternative therapies, methods of treatment used *instead* of orthodox medicine. I am totally and unequivocally opposed to any form of alternative treatments!

Sometimes you may hear a person describing a treatment as "unorthodox." In my opinion, that term should not be used. It merely indicates the person using it is unfamiliar with the treatment and trying to discourage its use even though it might be helpful to the particular patient. In fact, sometimes this term is applied to legitimate experimental therapy.

Fifty years ago, anyone being cured from cancer could only have done so with surgery. Therefore, to relatively few surgeons, any methods of treatment other than surgery, such as radiation, chemotherapy, relaxation or prayer are unorthodox. Oncologists know that this position is totally foolish. A few doctors with tunnel vision will call any treatments other than straight medical treatments unorthodox. This is only because they feel that they are imbued with all the knowledge in the world, and since they weren't taught this, it can't be good. My advice is to ignore the negative connotation of the word unorthodox whenever used. The idea is to get well, and if unorthodox methods can help, then after you are well you can try to figure out whether it was the orthodox or unorthodox treatments that did the most good.

The critical thing to differentiate between is alternative and supplemental treatments. Use your head and you will have no problem figuring out which is which. Everything recommended in this book is supplemental. It is in addition to whatever your qualified physician recommends.

Some people don't like the prospect of taking an unpleasant medical treatment. Perhaps some doctor told them there was nothing medically that could be done, and they failed to seek a second opinion. A human being will not be denied hope. They get oversold on a supplemental therapy, and use it to the exclusion of medical treatments. Then this supplemental therapy becomes an alternative therapy. It goes from something wonderful, something that can help save your life to something terrible, something that can most certainly cost you your life.

Ignore the word unorthodox, as it has no meaning other than to demean a particular treatment because it is not familiar. Stay far, far away from alternative therapies because they can kill you by denying you access to the treatments that thousands of scientists have developed and perfected over the years. Believe in and use every supplemental therapy that your physician says cannot hurt you. It is your life, and if you don't do everything possible to help yourself, no one else will.

There are numerous commonly used treatments for cancer, many of which could be successful if used individually, but often are proved more successful when used in combination. I personally had radiation therapy, chemotherapy, surgery, immunization therapy and a year of adjuvant chemotherapy in addition to psychotherapy. The cure rate for patients with advanced Hodgkin's disease was increased from 54% to 84% by giving alternating treatments with two four-drug combinations demonstrating the complexities within a single type of therapy. Different drugs are being used today but also in combination and in sequence, demonstrating the continuous advances in cancer treatments. We shall discuss several of the more common medical treatments.

We have all heard war stories about various treatments for cancer and how horrible they are. I had 5 of the more common treatments. Prior to that, I was told I was terminal, that nothing could be done and that there was no hope. I lived for 5 days without hope. I want to go on record as stating that any single minute without hope is worse than all the treatments I went through!

These horror stories were probably true in your parents' or grandparents' time. Today, these treatments, when administered by qualified professionals, are scientific, not guess work. They know exactly how much of anything can be given to you safely to do exactly what is supposed to be done and probably what the side effects or residual effects will be.

By far, the greatest progress in cancer treatments has been made in recent years. Over half of all cancers that a young doctor graduating from medical school only 20 years ago was taught were untreatable are today curable to some degree. At an annual review meeting of the National Cancer Advisory Board, Dr. Alan Rabson, then director of the Division of Cancer Biology and Diagnosis, referring to scientific highlights and discoveries, stated, "It has been one of the most exciting years during my lifetime." Dr. Lloyd Old of Memorial Sloan-Kettering, one of the most respected cancer specialists in the U.S., said there had been more progress made in the cancer field in the last several months than in the previous 25 years he had been in research. Dr. Vincent T. DeVita, Jr., former director of the National Cancer Institute, stated, "The pace at which science is moving is so exciting that the fear is not being able to keep up between the laboratory and the clinic."

People were burned with radiation therapy years ago. Today, there is no excuse for this. Sure, some people were poisoned with drugs. My recollection is that in an article a few years ago in the *Washington Post*, the reporter was able to locate some 6 drug-related deaths nationally. They showed a picture of an infant superimposed over her death certificate stating this child was killed by drugs. What dramatic journalism! These 6 deaths were out of some 200,000 people who received chemotherapy that year. If you compare the risk to the reward, there is no comparison. In my opinion, that article, by frightening people away from the proper treatment, killed more people than drugs would for many, many years.

Some 25 years ago a radical mastectomy was the treatment of choice for breast cancer. Now it is rarely an option. Relatively no one should die from testicular cancer today. Many say the greatest advances have been made in childhood cancers.

Be grateful that dedicated doctors and scientists discovered the treatments and perfected them so you are able to receive the benefits of them. Only a few years ago this was not possible. Because many people died previously, maybe you have a chance of beating cancer. Do everything your qualified doctor recommends to help save your life.

SURGERY: In a meeting at the National Cancer Institute, we were told that today surgery is given credit for 60% of those cured from cancer. Radiation therapy is credited for 25% and chemotherapy 15%. As you can see from these statistics, if you have a tumor that is surgically removable, your case has an optimistic outlook.

But don't get the wrong impression. First of all, not too many years ago surgery was the only possible treatment for cancer. Therefore, surgery's current cure rate of 60% is a reduction from 100% a short time ago.

Secondly, don't confuse inoperable with incurable. Maybe they sound somewhat alike, but they don't mean anything similar. I was inoperable and here I am writing this book. Inoperable means that at the moment, in the opinion of the doctor who is examining you, it cannot be operated on. It does not mean that you cannot be successfully treated without surgery. Also, it does not mean that other treatments could not make you operable. In my case, radiation and chemotherapy reduced the size of the tumor to make it operable. In addition, it does not necessarily mean that another surgeon with more experience or skills could not successfully perform the surgery.

Surgery, other than for taking a biopsy or debulking a tumor, is generally used in cancer treatment only when it can cure a patient or solve a particular problem, such as a stopped-up colon or ureter. Therefore, if surgery cannot be expected to completely cure a patient, it would not be considered the treatment of choice, and other options should be examined. There is no reason to debilitate the patient, postponing possibly curative treatments, for the sake of performing surgery.

Furthermore, in my personal opinion, while surgery is properly given credit for

60% of those cured from cancer, I believe that failure to give additional treatments prior to or following surgery is responsible for many of the deaths from cancer. That is why I urge every patient to receive a multi-disciplinary opinion prior to any treatment or to confirm with a board certified oncologist the surgeon's statement that no further treatments are necessary.

Since surgery is the treatment of choice in many cancers, the National Cancer Institute is directing a major expenditure for improving the use of surgery in cancer cases. At the beginning of a presentation on improving surgery, we were given a note of caution in the form of a quotation from an eminent surgeon: "There must be a final limit to the development of manipulative surgery. The knife cannot always have fresh fields for conquest and although methods of practice may be modified and varied, and even improved to some extent, it must be within a certain limit, that this limit has nearly if not quite been reached. It will appear evident if we reflect on the great achievements of modern operative surgery;

very little remains for the boldest to devise or the most dextrous to perform." This quote is from Sir John Erickson and was published in *Lancet*, a leading British medical publication on June 15, 1863!

CHEMOTHERAPY: Once the black sheep of cancer treatments, chemotherapy has become the leading weapon for increasing the number of patients who can be cured of cancer. At the same time, researchers are reducing the debilitating side effects that chemotherapy patients have typically had to endure.

"When chemotherapy was developed in the 1950's, cancer statistics were pretty much static," observed Dr. Bruce Chabner, former head of the National Cancer Institute's Division of Cancer Treatment. "Surgery had gone as far as it could go in curing local disease, and the radiation therapy of the 1960's and 1970's only improved the cure of local and regional disease.

"Unfortunately at the time of diagnosis, about half of cancer patients already have spread of their disease beyond their original site, and the only therapy that has made in-roads against these cancers is chemotherapy."

Now an additional 50,000 patients with cancer who cannot be cured by surgery or radiation are being saved each year by drug treatments. Fifteen years ago, chemotherapy cured just a few thousand patients annually. The future promise of chemotherapy is very bright. Recent discoveries of ways to improve the effectiveness of drugs and overcome resistance to them, as well as better understanding of how cancer cells spread to other parts of the body, are beginning to produce new treatment tactics that should further increase drug cures and extend chemotherapy to common cancers not currently vulnerable to its effect.

"The prognosis for patients with disseminated malignancy has improved considerably," Dr. Chabner said. Especially notable is the increase in long-term disease-free survival time for patients with testicular cancer from 10% in 1973 to 91% in 2002. Similarly, the response rate for patients with ovarian cancer has risen from 30% in 1973 to 95% in 2002. Further improvements in the efficacy of chemotherapy are expected to be attained with the refinement of high-dose chemotherapy, regional chemotherapy, bone marrow transplantation, the use of colony-forming assays to predict response, the use of combinations of noncross-resistant drugs, and the development of analogs of currently used agents.

The new chemotherapy approaches are increasing the damage done to cancer cells and diminishing effects on normal tissue. Chemotherapists are also better able to control the occasional side effects of nausea and vomiting. Currently, one patient in four who receive chemotherapy is cured!

The importance of drugs is universally acknowledged now that cancer specialists realize that the disease is often systemic, or bodywide, not confined to one site or tissue. In such cases, only treatments like drugs that can reach the nooks and crannies of the body wherever cancer cells may be hiding can be successful.

Cancer cells lose their ability to control their own growth. Normal cells know when to stop growing. If half of your liver is removed in an operation, for example, your liver will grow back. Once local repair is complete, growth stops.

Something happens to cancer cells so that they lose their ability to respond to the body's signal to stop growing. They become wild, erratic cells that keep multiplying.

By themselves, cancer cells are not usually destructive, but they keep proliferating in the body so that they eventually crowd out the normal tissue of organs. That's what kills the patient. If the cancer is in the lungs, for example, the eventual replacement of healthy tissues by malignant cells interferes with breathing.

Many of the new drugs and biological agents now being tested are aimed at controlling the growth of cancer cells rather than destroying them. In a sense, we want to give cancer cells the correct signal to stop growing and behave like normal cells.

The drugs fall into four main categories:

• Alkylating agents. The genetic material, or DNA, of a cell is made up of molecules, called bases, that must be duplicated and precisely paired when the cell divides. Alkylating agents interfere with the orderly pairing process and prevent successful division. Some of the prominent drugs in this family: Cytoxan and L-PAM.

- Antimetabolites. These compounds chemically resemble vitamins or other nutrients and are therefore absorbed by the cell. But once inside, they disrupt the cell's metabolic machinery. Such agents include methotrexate, 5-FU and 6-mercaptopurine (6-MP). 5-FU, for example, resembles uracil, a substance the cell needs to make DNA. It is not, however, a proper substitute and effectively blocks DNA synthesis.

- Antibiotics. Some of these were discovered in research for new drugs to fight infections. They disrupt the synthesis of RNA, a substance the cell needs to make essential proteins. Two leading antibiotics in cancer therapy: bleomycin and Adriamycin.

- Steroids. It isn't precisely known how these hormones, which include prednisone and estrogen, work against cancer. They are believed to prevent the production of proteins or other key enzymes.

- Some of the anti-cancer drugs don't fall into general categories. Vinblastine and vincristine, derived from the periwinkle plant, prevent the cell from doubling. The drug L-Alparaginase is an enzyme that destroys asparagine, an amino acid that some cancer cells can't make for themselves and must draw from the bloodstream. Normal cells, which synthesize the asparagine they need, are apparently unaffected by the drug.

ANTI-ANGIOGENESIS: These are drugs that block angiogenesis, the development of new blood vessels. Solid tumors cannot grow beyond the size of a pinhead (1 to 2 cubic millimeters) without inducing the formation of new blood vessels to supply the nutritional needs of the tumor. By blocking the development of new blood vessels, researchers are hoping to cut off the tumor's supply of oxygen and nutrients, and therefore its continued growth and spread to other parts of the body.'

A news article on the front page of the *New York Times* discussed research on the effects of angiostatin and endostatin (referred to as anti-angiogenesis) in treating cancer in mice. The article and subsequent coverage by other media generated intense public interest about these compounds. Dr. Judah Folkman and colleagues at Children's Hospital in Boston had reported data in the scientific journal *Nature* indicating that angiostatin and endostatin worked better in combination than either one alone in inducing regression of tumors in mice. It will possibly be an exciting treatment method in the future.

What we found so fascinating was that Dr. Folkman offered a bonus to any colleague who could find a tumor strain that was not affected by anti-angiogenesis. There were no winners! More than a dozen agents aimed at controlling or treating cancer by inhibiting tumor blood vessels now are being tested in clinical trials sponsored by drug companies and the National Cancer Institute.

Pharmaceutical companies announced that they are developing 316 new medicines to fight cancer including gene therapies, "magic bullet" antibodies, and light activated medicines, all new weapons in the high-tech, high stakes war against cancer.

Out of 1,000 laboratory-engineered chemical relatives of cis-platinum, the most potent of the recently developed chemotherapy agents, 2 have been found to retain their potency but have less severe side effects.

Many people expect worse side effects from chemotherapy than actually occur. Your doctor must, and rightfully so, warn you of all the possible side effects that have happened to anyone taking that particular drug. Many patients are able to work and perform most or all of their normal activities while receiving chemotherapy.

Does Cancer Chemotherapy Work?

HISTORICAL PERSPECTIVE:

Dioscorides (50-79 A.D.) used an extract of colchicum autumnale leaves soaked in wine to "dissolve tumors and growth."

Pliny (23-79 A.D.) and Ibn Sina (980-1037 A.D.) thought the extract worked, but Galen (129-210 A.D.) did not.

Abu Mansar (circa 977 A.D.) and Hildegaard (1098-1178 A.D.) thought it was more a poison than a medicine, because it caused nausea, vomiting, hair loss, and loss of appetite.

Today it is known that colchicine, its analogs, and the related vinca alkaloids are highly effective against certain hematologic malignancies.

RADIATION THERAPY: As a result of technical advances and training programs, radiation oncology has developed into a highly refined specialty. Now, with superb accuracy, a radiation beam can be focused on the tumor without damaging surrounding normal tissue. Linear accelerators, which hit tumors with up to 40 million electron volts, many times the dose of earlier machines, provide deeper penetration and a more precise beam that does less damage to healthy cells. By itself, as well as in combination with other therapies, radiation therapy is an increasingly potent tool.

Radiation therapy, in contrast to what many people imagine, does not destroy or dissolve cancer cells like a laser beam would. Possibly, if the dose were multiplied many, many times, it would. However, it is given in such small doses that its prime mission is to damage the DNA of a malignant cell. The cell does not die instantly, but when it tries to divide, it is unable to and dies at that time. Therefore, radiation treatments continue to be effective on the tumor after the treatments are completed, often for 90 days and more. Sometimes, tumors shrink primarily after the therapy is finished.

Radiation treatments are normally given 5 days a week, not because the doctors don't like to work on the weekends or have a strong union, but because during the other two days, normal healthy cells will repair the damage done to their DNA. Cancerous cells are unable to repair this damage.

Because scar tissue will continue to build up, changes could be noticed in follow up X-rays even though the tumor is gone. Also, no changes may be noticed in a bone scan for some time even though the radiation did its job because the bone mending itself after radiation will give the same image as a tumor on a scan.

IMMUNIZATION THERAPY: Some of the most exciting possibilities are offered by drugs that work in entirely different ways from the conventional ones. One such approach is immunotherapy, using drugs that cause the body's immune system to attack cancer just as it fights off infections.

The concept is based on two theories. First, cancer cells can be perceived by the immune system as "foreign" and, with proper help, rejected. The second is that cancer victims have lost their natural powers of rejection because of their debilitating disease.

The widely publicized drug, interferon, stemmed from immunological research. Discovered in the 1950's, it is a protein produced by body cells to help fight off viral infections. In cancer, researchers think it fastens onto cells and causes the release of enzymes that inhibit growth. And, because it is a natural substance, experts hope the side effects will be limited. So far, this is mostly theory; until recently, large scale testing of interferon hasn't been possible because it could be extracted only in minute quantities and at great cost from donated white blood cells. The emergence of recombinant DNA technology, in which common bacteria can be programmed genetically to manufacture quantities of proteins, has only recently made it possible to obtain enough interferon for cancer research.

On December 5, 1985, the *New England Journal of Medicine* carried a story on Dr. Steve Rosenberg's treatment of Interleukin II combined with LAK cells. That started a torrent of publicity throughout the winter of 1985-1986. Simply stated, this treatment took the natural killer cells from a patient's blood, treated them with IL-2, and reinjected them and more IL-2 back into the patient. These IL-2 armed white cells, called LAK or lymphokine-activated "killer cells," destroy tumors for months after administration in some cases, until the patient is clear of detectable cancer. Only patients who had failed all other treatments were accepted for this protocol. The success in reducing tumor burden by 50% or more was striking in several types of advanced cancer. In February, 1986, we received a report that Dr. Rosenberg had been successful in 100% (6 out of 6) of the cases of renal cell cancer and 50% (5 out of 10) of the cases of advanced malignant melanoma. Both of these types of cancers were relatively untreatable using other methods of treatment if surgery failed. Steps are underway to confirm and extend these results in other centers.

The most exciting aspect of this treatment, to me, is that IL-2 is not intended to harm the malignant cells. It is solely to stimulate the patient's own immune system which in turn destroys the cancer. Surgery, radiation or chemotherapy, the methods of treatment most physicians are used to discussing in fighting cancer, are each designed to damage malignant cells in their own way. The mere concept of IL-2, as well as the success of the treatments, emphasizes the importance of the patient's immune system. It throws wide open a new and separate field in fighting cancer.

It seems that there are a number of substances that occur naturally in the body to maintain normal growth and development which may be utilized to stimulate the body's natural defenses against cancer. The National Cancer Institute has established a special research program to explore intensively the therapeutic applications of these naturally occurring substances called "Biological Response Modifiers." In addition to IL-2 and interferon, this group includes thymosin, IL-1, IL-3, IL-4, IL-6, IL-12, tumor cell vaccines, tumor necrosis factor (TNF), etc.

HYPERTHERMIA: This is the process of heating a tumor approximately 10 degrees Fahrenheit. It is generally done with a microwave type mechanism. This in and of itself is capable of killing certain types of cancers. But that is not where the great promise lies. It has been found that hyperthermia can magnify the benefits of chemotherapy or radiation therapy several fold without much downside risk. A critical matter is monitoring the exact temperature of the tumor and the surrounding tissue. For this reason, it had previously been done on lesions relatively near the surface. However, great advances are being made, and it is being tried with many types of cancers. The moderate increase in temperature is not damaging to ordinary cells and not dramatically uncomfortable the patient. In many applications, hyperthermia is considered experimental today with tremendous potential. Hyperthermia is also often combined with radiation or chemotherapy.

HORMONAL MANIPULATION: The art of treating certain cancers by denying needed hormones, hormonal manipulation is normally one of the more pleasant treatments as it is non-toxic and has very minimal side effects. The possibility of its use is tested for regularly in breast cancer. If applicable, it is certainly a treatment of choice and can be used along with other forms of therapy. A pathologist described it in a fascinating way. A malignant cell is examined and found to be estrogen or progesterone positive, meaning it is dependent on those substances for survival. There is a door on the side of each malignant cell that opens to allow those substances to enter. By giving a certain pill, those doors are sealed shut and the malignant cells are deprived of this hormone they need to survive and divide and are killed.

DIE LASER: Also known as photodynamic therapy, it was developed at Roswell Park Memorial Institute in Buffalo, New York in the early 1970's. A non-toxic drug, Hpd, is injected and is absorbed only by malignant cells. It sensitizes these malignant cells to light. About three days later, an intense laser light is shined on the tumor for 8 to 10 minutes, producing high-powered singlet oxygen inside the cell so reactive that it burns up everything in sight, destroying the cancerous growth. Since the light can only penetrate 5 to 10 millimeters, it does not work well on treating thick or deep-seated tumors. It appears to work best on early to middle-stage cancers of the lung, bronchi and bladder. The use of die laser is increasing dramatically in many major cities, but it is still generally considered an experimental therapy.

MONOCLONAL ANTIBODIES: These are stirring great interest among researchers. The surfaces of viruses, bacteria and even normal cells contain specific molecules that are called antigens. When they enter the body, these molecules trigger certain blood cells to produce antibodies, proteins that lock onto the antigens and render them harmless. All vaccines are made from antigens that induce the formation of antibodies in advance to ward off infectious diseases.

First, researchers inject a mouse with an antigen — for example, a human cancer cell. The mouse then makes antibodies to different components of the cancer cell, including abnormal proteins associated with cancer itself. The investigator removes the mouse's spleen, where much of the antibody production occurs, and extracts its cells. They then fuse these cells with cancer cells from another mouse with myeloma. These tumor cells are used because they are immortal: they will continue to divide ad infinitum and make the fused hybrid do the same. Finally, the scientists select the hybrid cells that are producing the particular antibodies they want and encourage them to reproduce, or clone, in separate tissue cultures. All of this is done in the laboratory. The products are called monoclonal antibodies because each comes from a single line, or clone, of cells.

If special antigens can be found on cancer cells that are not present on normal cells, the lab-produced antibodies would home in on tumors like heat-seeking missiles while ignoring normal tissue. These antibodies could be tagged with radioactive substances or chemicals to carry lethal doses directly to cancer cells while bypassing normal cells.

Also, they have the potential of causing a revolution in diagnosis. Doctors can tag these antibodies with radioisotopes and scan the whole body for individual clusters of cancer cells that cannot be detected with current methods. While today they have been developed for only a few of the many types of cancer, and what has been developed is in extremely short supply compared to the demand, the entire concept of monoclonal antibodies is mind boggling and the potential is enormous.

CYTO-DIFFERENTIATORS: A new class of nontoxic drugs that render malignant cancer cells benign instead of killing them. In recent years, researchers discovered that normal cells, when very young, are much like cancer cells. They divide and spread rapidly and are undifferentiated — that is, without specific functions like skin or blood cells. If the young cell is disrupted, perhaps by a carcinogen, as it is growing toward the more mature, differentiated stage, it can become stuck in its immature phase, proliferating randomly and eventually forming a tumor.

GENE THERAPY: Gene therapy has a particular potential application to cancer because there is a strong genetic basis to many cancers. Cancers often grow and spread because of the mutations in their genes. The cancer cells' mutations may make them invisible to the immune system so they can't be rejected, or the mutations may take away the growth controls built into all cells, resulting in their uncontrolled growth. Gene therapy puts genes into cancer cells to make them stimulate the immune system or to restore growth control. Another approach is to put genes into the body's white blood cells to make them effective killers of the patient's cancer cells.

Gene therapy, at the present time, is considered to be highly experimental. All gene therapy treatments are part of scientific protocols which investigate the safety and side effects of the treatment as well as its effect on the cancer. All gene therapy protocols are also highly regulated in order to protect the patient participants. This includes a special committee of the National Institutes of Health called RAC (recombinant DNA advisory committee). It consists of doctors, scientists, ethicists, lawyers and lay people.

The most highly developed approach to cancer gene therapy is the use of gene-modified cancer cells as vaccines. Patients' tumors are removed, the cancer cells extracted, the genes are inserted and then the patients are immunized with their own gene-modified tumor cells. This approach works very well in animal models of gene therapy, but it is to be confirmed in human cancer.

Overall, gene therapy is a highly promising approach to cancer treatment but is experimental and unproven at the present time.

I would like to tell a story for the sake of the cancer patient looking for proper help. They say a picture is worth 10,000 words, and this brief story is a graphic picture. A friend was unexpectedly diagnosed with a very serious cancer of the sinuses at an outstanding institution. The surgeon who had done the biopsy and removed all the tumor mass possible originally, upon learning the cell pathology, stated that the only hope was for extremely radical surgery with pre-op or post-op radiation. The patient went to a second institution for a second opinion from a noted surgeon. There, he was told that radiation would not help and much more radical surgery than he had been led to expect would be necessary, nearly obliterating his face, if there was any hope of saving his life.

Being totally unnerved, he went back to the first institution for a consultation with the radiation therapist. Here, he was told that the surgery was far too dangerous and his only hope was in radiation therapy, which could be very damaging. Then, he went to a third institution where a medical oncologist, radiation therapist and surgeon sat down together with the patient after numerous additional tests were performed. Jointly, they worked out the possibility that a very low dose radiation could be given over 5 weeks fairly safely compared to the high dose that had been proposed, followed by surgery from the top of the head causing minimal appearance damage. However, the head and neck surgeon wanted a neurosurgeon present for that part of the operation.

I know none of this first hand. It has all been told to me by the patient and his wife directly. Maybe none of it is what he was told.

That doesn't make any difference. It is definitely what he understood. Obviously, he chose the latter institution. He chose the physicians who did not feel they knew more about other methods of treatments than the specialists in those methods. He wanted doctors who were open to the suggestions of others and who sought and wanted the assistance of specialists in fields other than their own. All this gave him hope which helped his mental attitude and gave him a strong desire to fight and live. The result of his search and the subsequent teamwork shrank the tumor with radiation to a point where it could be removed with adequate margins and no facial disfigurement.

———————

Articles in local publications or media announcing gigantic breakthroughs in cancer should be viewed with skepticism and not allowed to raise false hopes or doubts. Generally, these can be checked out easily by calling 1-800-4-CANCER, the Cancer Information Service at the National Cancer Institute. Major break-throughs, if publicly announced, would be important enough to make all the major wire services. You would hear about them on all the radio and TV news programs as well as in newspapers and magazines.

The following is from an article in *Good Housekeeping*, by Dr. Alan E. Nourse, about what you can do to avoid being taken in by cancer quackery.

"First, I think it is important to recognize what really is being done by modern medical science, slow as the progress may appear. Researchers are piecing together an immensely complicated puzzle, and progress is slow precisely because the puzzle is so intricate. To discover why a normal cell goes wrong and how to stop the process, we have to understand some of the most basic processes of life itself. But, bit by bit, the answers are coming in.

"Second, we should bear in mind that even though a 'magic bullet' against cancer may not be found, more and more kinds of cancer are being cured, and the list of known, effective treatments is lengthening.

"Third, knowing what we do about the dedication and integrity of most medical scientists, we should be suspicious of anyone who claims that researchers are deliberately hiding valid cancer cures from the public.

"But most important of all, we should use some plain good judgment. When you hear about a new cancer remedy that sounds simple and easy and that you can handle largely by yourself, recognize it for what it is. If it sounds too good to be true, it almost certainly *isn't* true."

STOP! Before reading any further, please answer the questions in the following quiz. It is meant, like everything else in this book, for your good and to help you fight cancer. If you read past this quiz before taking it, the quiz would be totally meaningless.

This test is not scientifically proven accurate. It is strictly a personal opinion after talking with many cancer patients as well as professionals. The questions have been reviewed by three teams of doctors, psychiatrists and psychologists in Kansas City, at Memorial Sloan-Kettering and at the National Cancer Institute. It is meant to enable you to assess your mental attitude and thus to help you successfully fight your disease.

In answering the questions, remember you are doing this for yourself. No one else ever

need see your answers. Do not put down what
you think you **should** say, put down what you
honestly **feel**. Do not try to figure out hidden
meanings. Answer each question quickly, as if
it were asked you in conversation.

Type of Cancer_____

Type of Cell _____

Date Diagnosed _____

✓ only	Treatment Received	Treatment Proposed
Surgery	_____	_____
Chemotherapy	_____	_____
Radiation	_____	_____
Immunization	_____	_____
Hyperthermia	_____	_____
Hormones	_____	_____
Psychotherapy	_____	_____

1. I feel that I have had more than my share of bad things happen to me.
   ❏ True   ❏ Unsure   ❏ Untrue

2. I am happy with my life and would like it to continue as it has been.
   ❏ True   ❏ Unsure   ❏ Untrue

3. I believe my cancer will get the best of me.
   ❏ True   ❏ Unsure   ❏ Untrue

4. I would do anything a nurse told me to do without questioning her.
   ❏ True   ❏ Unsure   ❏ Untrue

5. I have full faith in my doctor.
   ❏ True   ❏ Unsure   ❏ Untrue

6. I believe the treatment I am receiving will successfully treat me.
   ❏ True   ❏ Unsure   ❏ Untrue

7. If I were told to have an X-ray similar to one taken the previous day, I would do it without question.
   ❏ True   ❏ Unsure   ❏ Untrue

8. I do not want to discuss my cancer with my family.
   ❏ True   ❏ Unsure   ❏ Untrue

9. I do not want to discuss my cancer with my friends.
   ❏ True   ❏ Unsure   ❏ Untrue

10. If I had a trip, business meeting or other important occasion planned, I would postpone a doctor's appointment or treatment.
    ❏ True   ❏ Unsure   ❏ Untrue

11. There are certain treatments I would refuse even if the doctor said it was necessary.
    ❏ True   ❏ Unsure   ❏ Untrue

12. I believe I can beat cancer without the help of my doctor.
    ❏ True   ❏ Unsure   ❏ Untrue

13. If my doctor recommended a treatment I didn't like, I might try an alternative treatment such as Laetril.
    ❏ True   ❏ Unsure   ❏ Untrue

14. I prefer to know as little as possible about my treatments.
   ❑ True   ❑ Unsure   ❑ Untrue

15. I would not question my doctor or in any way hurt his feelings.
   ❑ True   ❑ Unsure   ❑ Untrue

16. I feel so nervous much of the time that I can't think very well.
   ❑ True   ❑ Unsure   ❑ Untrue

17. I feel so depressed most of the time that the future looks bleak to me.
   ❑ True   ❑ Unsure   ❑ Untrue

18. I have had serious emotional problems in the past that are now kicking up again.
   ❑ True   ❑ Unsure   ❑ Untrue

You are finished with the questions. Now take a blank sheet of paper and score your results. If the type of cancer is blank or unknown, score 10 points. If the type of cell is blank or unknown, score 5 points.

Under treatment received, if no treatment has been received, score 10 points if diagnosed 60 days ago and 5 points if diagnosed 30 days ago. If currently malignant and no treatment is being received or proposed, score 10 points.

1.	5 True	2 Unsure		
2.		2 Unsure	10 Untrue
3.	15 True	2 Unsure		
4.	5 True	2 Unsure		
5.		2 Unsure	5 Untrue
6.		2 Unsure	5 Untrue
7.	5 True	2 Unsure		
8.	5 True	2 Unsure		
9.	5 True	2 Unsure		
10.	5 True	2 Unsure		
11.	10 True	2 Unsure		
12.	15 True	2 Unsure		
13.	5 True	2 Unsure		
14.	5 True	2 Unsure		
15.	10 True	2 Unsure		
16.	5 True	2 Unsure		
17.	5 True	2 Unsure		
18.	5 True	2 Unsure		

Add 5 points for 5 or more "unsure."

Total all your points. A score of 25 or less indicates your attitude is favorable. A score above 25 indicates that you should consider help. The first step is to get recommendations. Talk to your doctor, clergyman, family or friends to suggest a psychiatrist, psychologist or other person who is experienced in counseling cancer patients. Arrange a consultation and be certain you have a good rapport with and confidence in the person. Follow the program they advise, especially as it relates to working with your medical doctors and cooperating in your treatments.

If you scored badly, don't assume that it doesn't apply to you or, now that you know the answers, you will change. Questions are merely indicative of the fundamentals and are from more than 100 that could have been used.

Let's discuss the questions individually and the logic behind each. Not only might you understand some aspects that cancer specialists feel give a better chance of success, but you may pick up specific ideas you had not thought of to help yourself fight cancer.

On the type of cancer and type of cell, if you left either blank or don't know, it could indicate that you lack interest and are failing to take your cancer seriously or do not desire to educate yourself. Either of these are unfavorable signs. I have talked with people who do not know whether they had lung, colon or pancreas cancer. Their doctor told them they were malignant, and they did not want to know any more. This is a form of denial, as if you buried your head in the sand, it might go away. The type of cell is important to know because you should understand as much as possible about your disease to cooperate with your physician in treatments. It is more technical than the type of cancer, so it only scores 5 points instead of 10.

Occasionally, the primary (site of origin) cannot be found. If this is after looking at all the areas from which the cell could have originated without success along with qualified second opinions, it is possible the prognosis is better than many known primaries. However, cancer cannot be efficiently and simply treated with maximum aggressiveness without knowing the specific primary. Therefore, every reasonable effort should be made to locate the primary. After you have exhausted all second opinions locally without success or agreement, you should suggest to your pathologist that he send your slides to the Armed Forces Institute of Pathology in Washington, D.C. Operated by the U.S. government, their services are completely free. They have equipment that is state-of-the-art and often superior to what is available in parts of the U.S. They have an information desk open 24 hours a day at (202) 576-2800.

If no treatment has been received within 30 days of diagnosis, it can indicate that you are not recognizing the critical nature of cancer and the fact that it is probably never as treatable as it is right now. Most cancers are treatable at the time they are discovered. If they go untreated properly, at some time in the future — whether tomorrow, next month or next year — they will be untreatable. If you've let it go 60 days, obviously the situation is more serious.

If you have a malignancy and no treatment is being given or recommended, you are a masochist and intentionally are waiting for it to get worse, or you have not exhausted all your options and are waiting to die. As a California oncologist told me, there are always options for treatments. As long as he had been practicing, he had never seen a patient run out of possibilities for treatment as long as they were alive.

Questions 1 and 2 are two different ways of attempting to determine your subconscious will to live. If you feel that you have more than your share of bad things happen or if you would not like your life to continue as it has, you probably are not fighting as hard as possible to continue living.

Question 3 is one of the two most critical questions on the quiz. It comes from the theory expressed by many oncologists that there is no way to cure a person who thinks they will die from their cancer. If a person thinks they will die, they are right. That is not to say that if a person thinks they will recover, they will, but at least they have a chance. My personal opinion is that if you have answered question 3 true, you need counseling without regard to any other part of the test because subconsciously you have thrown in the towel and only a miracle could save you.

Question 4 is not intended to be derogatory to a nurse. It merely indicates that you are not taking an interest in trying to educate yourself and help your body help the treatments that fight your disease.

A negative reply to question 5 or 6 would indicate that not only don't you believe in your treatment, but you are probably taking the lazy way out by not searching for a qualified doctor who believes he can successfully treat you and in whom you have complete confidence.

Question 7 is a subtle way to ask if you believe you are in charge. This could be true of a blood test or anything else. This is your body. You are responsible for it. You should not necessarily have the same test two days in a row, but you should understand why it is needed and not allow anything to be done to you if it is not necessary.

Eight and 9 are critical questions, not only concerned with the successful treatment of your cancer but with the possibility of recurrence. Discussing your cancer is a necessity to vent your feelings and reduce stress. You should be willing to discuss your cancer openly, not incessantly. Failure to openly communicate will drive away your family or friends and eliminate an absolutely necessary ingredient of your support system. This is one factor I recognize most commonly in patients, one that can be most easily corrected because it is based on erroneous assumptions that those who want to help you don't want to be inflicted with your problems. In reality, they want to share your feelings because in this way they can sincerely express their love and devotion for you. We each have a need to be loved and nurtured. When ill, this need increases. Intimacy and affection can play a major role in healing.

Ten, 11, and 13 are a subtle way of asking your order of priorities. If you are anxious to be successfully treated but only if it is convenient for you, then you do not want it enough to give it your best shot. The same question could have been asked in many ways, such as, if you are a smoker, have you quit? To validate the severity of question 10, an oncologist stated he felt that the rhythm of the treatments, the timing, the fact that each

One Day at a Time

There are 2 days in every week about which you should not worry; days which should be kept free from fear and apprehension.

One of these days is YESTERDAY with its mistakes and cares, its faults and blunders, its aches and pains. Yesterday has passed forever beyond our control. All the money in the world cannot bring back yesterday. We cannot undo a single act we performed, we cannot erase a single word said. Yesterday is Gone!

The other day we should not worry about is TOMORROW, with its possible burden, its large promise and poor performance. Tomorrow is also beyond our immediate control. Tomorrow's sun will rise, either in splendor or behind a mask of clouds — but it will rise. Until it does, we have no stake in tomorrow, for it is yet unborn.

This leaves only one day — TODAY! Any man can fight the battle of just one day. It is only when you and I have the burdens in these two awful extremities — Yesterday and Tomorrow — that we break down.

It is not the experience of today that drives men mad; it is the remorse or bitterness about something which happened yesterday and the dread of what tomorrow will bring.

**LET US THEREFORE LIVE
BUT ONE DAY AT A TIME.**

treatment is given on schedule could be as important as what drugs are given. Eleven is valued greater because it is the person you have selected to treat you telling you that you need something specific, and you are going against that advice. I have heard patients say they would do anything except take radiation or chemotherapy or have surgery. What they are saying is that their mind is closed and they want to get well but not enough to do something unpleasant or frightening. They definitely won't give recovery their best effort.

Question 12 is the other single most important question. It embodies many unexpressed inferences. Anyone who believes they can beat cancer without the help of their physician is in a very dangerous predicament in my opinion. Some of the things it could imply are that you have no faith in the physician you chose, and therefore that you have no confidence in anything you are doing, including treatments. It may go further and imply that you have no faith in the medical system or in science. You may have an unrealistic confidence or unattainable expectations in spontaneous remission, spiritualism or alternative therapies. These are wonderful when used as an adjunct to orthodox medicine, but they are suicide when used in lieu of medicine.

Question 14 is fairly obvious on the surface. It is believed by many that understanding each treatment and exactly what it does to and for you will enhance that treatment and magnify its benefits. Closing your mind to these potential benefits indicates moderation of your desire to recover.

Number 15 is a great deal like 7 but on a much more direct and critical basis. This is your life. Your doctor is not God. If there is something you want to know, you should ask. If there is something you don't feel is right, you must express yourself. Your physician wants it this way. When a patient says to me that they would rather die than hurt their doctor's feelings, I say they will.

Sixteen, 17 and 18 are straight forward questions that indicate the state of your mental or emotional health. Often, they go unasked by your physician in the haste of meeting an appointment schedule. If nervousness, depression or emotional problems are present, not only can they depress the immune system in helping to fight your cancer or diminish the effects of many common treatments, but they can occupy your mind and hinder you from applying all your energy toward recovery.

The addition of 5 points for 5 or more unsure answers is based on the idea that strongwilled, decisive or determined people have a better chance of beating cancer. To put it in reverse, the wishy-washy, sweet, mild-mannered person does not have as good a chance. Saying you are not sure of your answer to 5 or more questions could indicate you fall in this latter category.

None of these factors are indisputable. There are exceptions. Also, none of your feelings on any subject are irreversible. However, the goal of this quiz is not to get you to change your opinion on any single question. It is to find out your attitude as it relates to being receptive to successful treatments for your cancer. If it is good, marvelous. Cooperate with your physician and let's get on with fighting cancer. If it is on the wrong side of 25, which in and of itself is no magic number but merely an indication, let's do something about it. Talk to your doctor, your clergyman, your family or friends to get the recommendation of a counselor who is experienced in working with a cancer patient. It is another thing that can improve your percentages.

Mental Attitude 5

To quote from *The Healing Family*, "Cancer is a serious crisis — but isn't life a matter of adapting to one change after another? I believe we must continually adapt to survive, and as life goes on, we can thrive on living. There's no reason we cannot maintain a fine quality of life during a life-threatening crisis. The diagnosis of cancer is not an automatic death warrant that demands that the patient and his family stop living."

A study found that people participating in a fitness program were less depressed and anxious. Physical fitness has a direct and positive impact on psychological health. One should not rush into strenuous exercise, but it is not necessary to assume that some physical exercise is out of the question. By talking with your physician and possibly working with a

READ OUT LOUD DAILY

I realize the power within me is greater for me than the power of another. That I have the power to control my thoughts and that my thoughts control my feelings and the way I see the world around me.

I realize that negative thoughts create negative experiences and positive thoughts create positive experiences. Therefore I now decide to control my thoughts and think of the positive good side of me and my world.

I realize that thoughts dominant in my mind will manifest themselves in reality. Therefore I now decide to keep before me a positive, happy picture of my success.

I realize the spoken word is the most powerful. Therefore I speak good thoughts out loud and count my blessings out loud daily. I focus my thought energy on the good of me, of you, of today, of life.

I start my day by getting myself up.
I am glad to be alive. I love myself.
I feel wanted, needed, important, special.
This is the greatest day of my life!
I have joy and love in my heart!
I am eager to be here today and to give today that which I am!
No one is exactly like me!
I expect people to be glad to see me!

physical therapist, a cancer patient often can do a great deal of exercise resulting in the improvement of both his emotional and physical condition. Ohio State University found that exercise helped 93% of 251 cancer patients feel better physically and mentally.

Cancer victims who express emotions — especially their anger — and who seek support to help them cope with the disease fare better than those who adopt a stoic attitude and suppress their emotions, new studies show.

Among the breast cancer patients, those who were listless, apathetic and who withheld anger had more recurrences of cancer than patients who sought social and emotional support and expressed anger and other feelings.

Among skin cancer patients, those who subsequently died of their disease or had it spread and worsen, were more likely to have been depressed, emotionally withdrawn and silently hostile than those who had no recurrence of the disease up to three years after surgery.

The will to live is in itself an energy. It is a desire to fight for life because there is honestly something to live for. The shock and uncertainty of diagnosis cause many people to lose this and suspend living for a few weeks. This will to live will be stronger in patients who find their lives enjoyable and who have things in their lives they honestly look forward to.

One doctor stated, "About 15 to 20 percent of people who are seriously ill would prefer to die if given the opportunity, 50 to 60 percent are willing to get better so long as the doctor does the work and the medicine doesn't taste too bad. The final 15 to 20 percent say, 'I'll do anything I have to do to get well. Just show me.'" It is these latter people for whom this book is written.

This same doctor states that there is no danger in giving false hope because "there is no such thing as false hope...it's never therapy that heals, it's people who heal, and the best role for doctors is to encourage that healing process, to help some of the 50 to 60 percent who want the doctor to do all of the work to move over into the realm of the survivors."

Commitments for future activities can produce a powerful energy. Great results can come about from working toward meaningful goals. Family members should set goals for the patient and encourage plans for the future.

The low self-esteem confirmed by so many studies of cancer patients immediately begins to rise when they are encouraged to be selfish and express their anger. Once a patient becomes "I" oriented and emotionally expressive, they can make progress in their life and their healing.

The reason it is so important for a cancer patient to develop a more fulfilling, less stressful emotional life is that chronic depression and stress depress the immune response. Drugs and therapies are probably not as effective against cancer as the specific antigens an individual's body can create. Isolation increases depression and anxiety and can work against healing. A recent study showed people who had pets or plants to care for recuperated faster than those who didn't. Living things that depend upon us for survival give us a purpose and a feeling of being needed.

Make it a point to set aside time every day for your own pleasure. This can be anything from a sport or playing cards or talking on the phone or going to a movie. The important thing is to break your normal routine just for the sake of doing something that gives you pleasure. The mere act of doing something exclusively for your own benefit is good therapy.

Outside support is essential to a cancer patient. Talking your feelings over with someone allows you to feel them fully and helps release them. There are numerous ways support can be established: through your physician, your church, your office, your team sport or a self help group. Stress management becomes crucial with the diagnosis of cancer. Exercise, relaxation, recreation and expression of feelings are ways to relieve stress.

You cannot begin to deal with stress until you realize and admit that you are under stress. Until you reach that point, you will not successfully cope with it. The mere diagnosis of cancer places a large burden of stress not only on you, but on your family and friends, which in turn adds to your stress. It is important to analyze what you are doing to adjust your priorities and responsibilities. Avoid taking on any unnecessary responsibilities during your recovery. Your goal must be to reduce stress, and this must be accomplished not only with all the positive actions, but by avoiding taking on any additional factors that could increase stress. Examples would be going in debt for a major purchase or trip because you "may not" have much time left, or getting married when you had not planned to but felt you "must" because of the circumstances.

Physician-Patient Communication   6

The two most common complaints with all cancer patients are fear of the unknown and failure of communication with their doctor. These are both absolutely normal, and no one is to blame. The doctor doesn't know what the patient is afraid of or wants to know, and the patient, having never been there, doesn't know what to ask. Furthermore, often the patient does not hear what the doctor says.

Since this book is being written for you, there are two specific things you can do to improve communications between you and your physician. First, whenever you are with your doctor, not only should you have a friend or family member present to help ask the questions and understand the answers, but you should have a tape recorder so that you can play it back at a later time when you can concentrate on what was said and not be under stress. No physician should object to a tape recorder because that is like saying he is not honest and would not want to admit what he said. If the physician is concerned with a potential lawsuit, he may want to have his own recorder operating simultaneously to avoid the possibility of an edited tape.

Secondly, you can nicely and politely but firmly insist that your doctor spend sufficient time with you to thoroughly answer all your questions and explain what may lie ahead of you between now and the time of your next visit. For this purpose, it is best that you have all your questions written out so that you can hand them to your doctor. This will save your rambling, repeating and omitting what you want to know. It will also let your doctor answer them all in a logical sequence in the time he has.

Important to recovery is your doctor's way of communicating with you about your disease. Many physicians now believe that if they instill a sense of confidence and hope in their patients, these patients will do better. A physician can easily communicate negativity to a patient by what he says, tone of voice or even line of sight. When a doctor dejectedly says, "There's not much more that we can do," you're likely to feel helpless. If you are told that despite the seriousness of your illness, there are treatments for it and one of them might improve your condition, the physician can still remain honest without dashing your spirits.

An article in *The New England Journal of Medicine* states that, "According to surveys, at least 70% of doctors now believe in telling people the truth about their cancers, as compared with 82% who practiced oppositely only 24 years ago."

It further advises physicians, "To begin, if you take time to talk with people, not at them, your story will be heard...One session may not be enough. Doctors who wish to retain more than 5% of a lecture's content must go over its material more than once — preferably soon, and again after a day — so why not patients?... You shouldn't tell more than you know. Admissions of ignorance confirm your knowledge. A patient or family member may ask you to peer into the future... you may wish to guess, extrapolate from what has gone on or invoke prior experience...resist if you can.

"Matter-of-factness is crucial. Pity and sympathy are distancing; they separate the giver from the receiver by emphasizing the differences in their lots. People in desperate trouble need sharing instead, which they get from the acknowledgment in your words of what they are up against, the promise in your attentiveness that you'll be there, and the declaration in your attitude that you and they are fellow wayfarers...

"Most important, keep people in charge. To usurp the role is tempting for either a physician or family member, but it will be one of a physician's less noble acts.

"The alternative to the approach of sharing the burden while promoting independence is to decide for oneself or with the family what to do. It often means complicated lying. Sometimes it means deciding to forgo treatment for someone entitled to make that decision. Worse, it means arrogating to oneself or a family member the decision about how someone will face death, and in the process making him or her subordinate and childlike. And it means saying things that inevitably will be contradicted by events, bringing an increasing portion of isolation and mistrust to someone who, more and more, will need their opposites. It must be especially hard to decline while everyone, including oneself, pretends it's not happening, or that it is for reasons too dreadful to be discussed.

A DOCTOR'S PRAYER
Before Giving a Prognosis to a Cancer Patient

Allow me to think about the ramifications
of my words before I give a prognosis
to a cancer patient. Because I have seen
others fail, do not let me deny this
individual the right to fight. Because I
have tried unsuccessfully with others, do
not let me condemn this person to a
sentence of hopelessness and
helplessness until he succumbs. Because
I am personally unaware of any
treatments that could give him any relief,
do not allow me to assume that there are
none nor deny him the right to search.
Help me use the intelligence and
compassion that was given to me and
help him search out the best
possible resources.

"I would make four points. The first is that we doctors are not wise enough to tell in advance who should not be told. We sense who would be difficult to tell, but that is a different matter, having as much to do with ourselves as our patients.

"The second point is that shielding is ultimately impossible and that the price of its temporary achievement is an enduring sense of betrayal. Once lied to, even supposedly in their own interest, people will not trust fully again. And the lie is inevitably discovered.

"The third is that even if we knew whom to shield and could carry it off, we still should not. Not only is lying wrong in an abstract sense, though one may argue over possible exceptions, but in this instance it is especially so.

"Finally, we physicians need to look further into ourselves, and to ask, when we falter at telling bad news or manage its consequences badly, how often it is a blinking at our own mortality, a reluctance to admit the failure of what we have done for prevention or cure, or an unworthy desire to control...

We should refer those patients...whose symptoms or diseases are beyond our competence."

A "Bill of Rights" for cancer patients and their physicians may help pave the way for an improved patient-oncologist relationship. It was prepared for the Wellness Community in cooperation with a group of practicing oncologists and is advocated by the UCLA Cancer Center. If you have a problem communicating with your oncologist, you might show this to him and ask him to abide by it, providing you agree to do your share.

As your physician, I will make every effort to:

1. Provide you with the care most likely to be beneficial to you.

2. Inform and educate you about your situation and the various treatment alternatives. How detailed an explanation is given will be dependent upon your specific desires.

3. Encourage you to ask questions about your illness and its treatment. I will answer your questions as clearly as possible. I will

also attempt to answer the questions asked by your family; however, my primary responsibility is to you, and I will discuss your medical situation only with those people authorized by you.

4. Remain aware that all major decisions about the course of your care shall be made by you. However, I will accept the responsibility for making certain decisions if you want me to.

5. Assist you to obtain other professional opinions if you desire, or if I believe it to be in your best interest.

6. Relate to you as one competent adult to another, always attempting to consider your emotional, social, and psychological needs as well as your physical needs.

7. Spend a reasonable amount of time with you on each visit unless required by something urgent to do otherwise, and give you my undivided attention during that time.

8. Honor all appointments unless required by something urgent to do otherwise.

9. Return phone calls as promptly as possible, especially those you indicate are urgent.

10. Make test results available promptly if you desire such reports.

11. Provide you with any information you request concerning my professional training, experience, philosophy, and fees.

12. Respect your desire to try treatments that might not be conventionally accepted. However, I will give you my honest opinion about such unconventional treatments.

13. Maintain my active support and attention throughout the course of the illness.

I hope that you as the patient will make every effort to:

1. Comply with our agreed-upon treatment plan.

2. Be as candid as possible with me about what you need and expect from me.

3. Inform me if you desire another professional opinion.

4. Inform me of all forms of therapy you are involved with.

5. Honor all appointment times unless required by something urgent to do otherwise.

6. Be as considerate as possible of my need to adhere to a schedule to see other patients.

7. Attempt to make all phone calls to me during regular working hours. Call on nights and weekends only when absolutely necessary.

8. Attempt to coordinate the requests of your family and confidants, so that I do not have to answer the same questions about you to several different persons.

The cancer patient, as well as the entire family, should attempt to live a life as close to normal as you feel comfortable. To allow for no changes is unrealistic because it denies the stress of living with a life-threatening disease. But the opposite, to curl up and quit enjoying life, is equally bad. Even with the toughest treatments, there is generally plenty of time for relaxation and pleasure. And each family member should not feel so indispensable that they cannot take time off for their own needs. As a result, they will be able to be of more benefit to the patient.

A woman was diagnosed with lung cancer. In spite of having a very devoted husband, extremely supportive children, a well-qualified medical oncologist and radiation oncologist, and no possible financial problems, she made no personal efforts to fight the disease. Sure, she took the prescribed radiation. But she never gave up smoking! She would not read anything about her problem or try to help herself. Then, as the disease worsened, she finally confided in her son why she acted the way she did. She said she was told after her initial chest X-ray by the diagnostic radiologist that she obviously had lung cancer. She should do whatever she wanted for whatever time she had left. She should not listen to anyone who wanted to help her because there was nothing that really would help!

Maybe that is what the radiologist said and maybe it isn't. It is what the patient thought she heard! In World War II, there was a saying, "Loose talk costs lives." The same words are even more applicable to cancer. There is much evidence — scientific, clinical and anecdotal — showing that a patient's expectations have a real bearing on the effectiveness of treatments. A health professional, doctor, nurse or technician has no right to make a statement from ignorance or one that can be misunderstood by the patient.

The following **"Physician/Patient Statement of Mutual Commitment"** should be shown to the primary physician treating your cancer at the earliest possible meeting. It should be discussed and agreed to. Unilaterally assuming each will do it anyway is taking a chance. Making the mutual commitment increases the likelihood of success.

Cancer is a complex disease with numerous treatment options. Often there is only one opportunity for success. Effective treatment requires effort by both the patient and physician. A clear understanding of what each can expect of the other will help. Thoughts and feelings of the doctor are transmitted neurologically, affecting the health of the patient.

Patient Commitment:

1. I will do everything in my power to assist in my healing.

2. I will keep all my appointments on time, listen attentively and follow the agreed-upon treatment to the letter.

3. I will keep you informed of any problems or questions.

4. I will keep you informed of any therapy or medications I take.

5. I will let you know about my concerns or worries that may affect my medical condition.

6. I will consciously choose to believe in <u>our</u> ability to make a difference in the healing process.

5. I will let you know about my concerns or worries that may affect my medical condition.

6. I will consciously choose to believe in <u>our</u> ability to make a difference in the healing process.

Physician Commitment:

1. I will be honest with you in stating facts, and optimistic when sharing judgment. (I will not state as a fact anything I do not know to be a fact.)

2. I will work with you to discover the very latest information known in my specialty for your particular disease and to identify medical and community information sources beyond my specialty.

3. I will not speak for any discipline other than my own. If I am uncertain, I will refer you to a qualified physician who might help.

4. I will listen attentively, and give sufficient time to courteously answer all your questions, in order that I might treat the "whole person."

5. I will respect your right to make an informed decision and abide by it.

6. I will consciously choose to believe in <u>our</u> ability to make a difference in the healing process.

Self Help Exercises   7

An *American Health* magazine article states, "How you feel about yourself affects your physical well-being. Researchers now recognize that a sense of purpose, a positive outlook and the feeling of being in control of one's life may help prevent illness, from cancer to the common cold.

"The notion that attitudes affect health is almost as old as medicine. But it's taken the re-emergence of certain humanistic values in medicine for doctors to put science to work charting exactly how the mind influences the body and vice versa.

"They are finding that attitude and state-of-mind can alter the responsiveness of nerve cells to a variety of chemicals that relay messages throughout the brain and nervous system. Further, chemical messengers of mood and motivation in the brain communicate with cells in the immune system responsible for countering invasion by tumors and microorganisms...

"It may be a long time before anyone draws a complete picture of the mind's effect on the body. But this much is known: we each have a larger role than ever imagined in combatting illness."

The body has an immune system. One of the theories is that part of the immune system is the thymus gland located in your chest directly behind the breast bone. The thymus gland has two specific functions. First of all, it creates 12 to 15 different hormones. These hormones travel throughout the body looking for cancer cells.

When they find the type of cell that they recognize, they do not harm the cell but attach themselves to it and send back a signal to the thymus gland. In response to this signal, the thymus gland dispatches a natural killer cell (NK cell) that goes directly to this hormone and kills the cell. It then returns to the thymus gland ready to be sent out again.

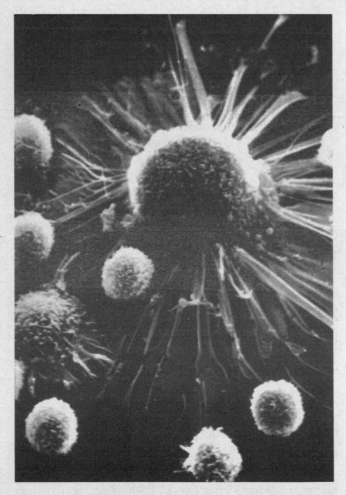

"Actual photograph of Natural Kill (NK) cells starting to attack a malignant cell."

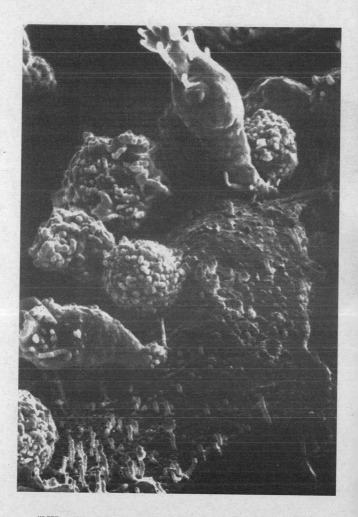

"NK cells in the process of destroying malignant cell."

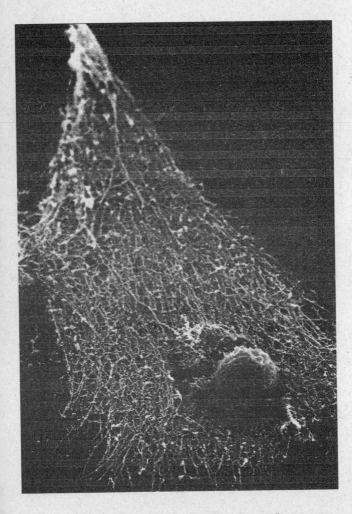

"NK cells leaving dead malignant cell."

One thought is that the thymus gland can be controlled by the brain in that during a time of trauma or depression, the brain will reduce the function of the thymus gland. During this period of reduced function, cancer cells, which are supposed to occur normally in each person some six times a year, are allowed to divide and multiply. When the trauma or depression is over, the thymus gland will resume normal operation. By this time, the cancer has had a chance to multiply and establish itself to the point where the NK cells are incapable of destroying it. At this point, we have cancer.

Two cancer treatment specialists rationalized that if the mind played a function in causing cancer, why couldn't the mind be trained to help treat the cancer. They started a clinic in 1976 and brought 150 cancer patients there. These were not normal cancer patients, though. They had two unique qualities. First, they were terminal because their doctor said they were going to die from their cancer. Second, they could have no possible medical treatments such as chemotherapy, surgery, radiation, hyperthermia, immunotherapy, etc. These people were going to die from their cancer.

They taught these people two things. First, they taught these people to relax. Not just superficially, but a way down deep relaxation. It is a scientifically proven fact that tumors grow faster in mice under stress. What is the dangerous part about your cancer? The fact that it will continue to grow! If your cancer never grew from where it is, you could live for another 100 years with it. If, by relaxing, you could slow down the growth of your tumor, you would be better off.

Second, they taught these people to visualize their cancer and think it away. Sound silly? Some two years later, when Annette and I read about them in the newspaper, of the initial group of 150 terminal cancer patients using only their minds to think away the cancer, some 10% were totally free of cancer. Another approximately 10% were dramatically improved. A third 10% had their cancer stabilized. My wife and I made up our minds that if I had a 30% chance of staying alive instead of none, we were going to go there. As it was, the doctors felt that they could successfully treat me. However, I used the relaxation and imagery in conjunction with the medical treatments. I cannot say that it is what cured me, but I can state without any question that it made me feel better. I believe it helped, and I positively know it did not hurt me. I would never recommend this in lieu of medicine, but only in addition to everything else your doctor wants you to do.

A study of 45 elderly residents in retirement homes suggests relaxation therapy may enhance a person's natural ability to fight disease. The study, conducted by researchers at Ohio State University, found an increase in cells that defend against viral infections and a decrease in certain antibody levels in volunteers who practiced relaxation techniques, compared to no change in control volunteers who didn't use the techniques.

In discussing these theories with doctors, I have found that those outstanding physicians whose primary interest is the recovery of the patient, who insist on an independent second opinion, who seek help from major cancer centers and refer their patients to qualified specialists, are staunch believers in this form of therapy in addition to medicine. The practitioners who are trying to build their practice generally have a desire to receive full credit for a cure without having to share it with any other institution, physician or method of therapy. Their most espoused argument against relaxation and imagery is that the statistics are inaccurate because the people who use it have a stronger desire to live than the average person. My answer is that I only want to help those who have a strong desire to live. If a person wants to die, that is their business. Those who want to live should have every opportunity to do so.

Occasionally, a shallow thinking health professional says that medical treatments are the only thing that cure cancer. He does not want his patient confused with the idea that anything but his doctor can help treat him. Mental attitude has nothing to do with it. Furthermore, if the patient tries mental imagery and it doesn't help them, they will have a guilt complex and that attitude will hinder their recovery. If that isn't talking out of both sides of their mouth, I don't know what is! If the patient's mental attitude could hinder their recovery, how could it have nothing to do with their recovery?

When someone can explain spontaneous remission to me, I'll quit believing in lots of things. The head of a major cancer center, an outstanding oncologist, told me he strongly believes in, as he put it, the will to live. He had a very good personal friend admitted with advanced cancer. He believed she had only a week or so to live. She was in critical condition. She had a daughter's wedding scheduled for some months hence and her husband had promised her a trip to Europe after the wedding. He urged her to move the daughter's wedding to the next few days because of her condition. She insisted she would make the wedding and the trip to Europe. Sure enough, she went into remission, was there to watch her daughter get married and even went on a wonderful trip to Europe feeling good. On the return trip, her cancer recurred. She returned directly to the hospital where she died a few days later.

Going even further, and this is a giant step further, Dr. Herbert Benson, the cardiologist who heads behavioral medicine at Boston's Beth Israel Hospital, one of the main teaching facilities at Harvard Medical School says, "Belief is the hidden ingredient in Western medicine and every traditional system of 'healing' I know about...A new drug given by a doctor who believes in it enthusiastically is far more potent than the same drug given by a skeptical doctor...Clinical studies have shown that a patient's belief in a medicine can make it far more effective."

From these comments, you can appreciate my statement that there are 3 fundamental requirements for an individual to have a chance to beat cancer. First is an honest, strong desire to live. Second is total confidence in their doctor. Third is absolute confidence that the treatment their doctor is recommending will successfully treat them. If any of these three factors is missing, I urge the patient to make a few telephone calls to see if a qualified physician can be found who can make them possible.

I have a stronger reason to believe this than anyone else. After being told I was terminal, I went to a doctor who said he would cure me. He did not say he would try this or hope for that. He said he would cure me, and he told me step by step exactly what would happen to me over the next year. Everything happened as he said it would and at the end of two years, I was cured. A year later, I heard an outstanding oncologist say there was no chemotherapy effective against my type of cancer. I felt like standing up and saying, "Here I am." Again, in 1984, some 6 years after these drugs helped cure me, I heard the head of a cancer center say the same thing. Then and only then, I realized what it probably was. Drugs alone are in truth probably ineffective against this type of cancer. But these same drugs, given by an enthusiastic physician to a patient who believes they will work and who practices mental imagery along with the drugs, did their intended job.

In other words, for some patients with cancer, there are no medical options. Relaxation and imagery could help in these cases. It positively cannot hurt. In most cases there are multiple medical options. Here, relaxation and imagery could help doubly by stirring up the body's own immune system to help kill the cancer, along with magnifying the effects of the treatments to destroy the cancer.

An additional benefit of relaxation and imagery is that it allows a patient to be intimately involved in their own recovery. It gives them a feeling of being at least partially in charge of their own destiny, which can do nothing but improve the quality of life. As the child of a patient so aptly put it in a letter, it made her father fight to live rather than wait to die.

Step-By-Step Methods

Relaxation and imagery, as the name implies, is a two-step process. It is felt that imagery can be much more effective only after relaxation has been successfully established. Relaxation is not a state of being that you hope or wish for; it is the result of a specific set of physical acts. If you follow the prescribed recommendations, you will end up relaxed. Several methods are suggested.

Some people are more receptive to one method than another. Try each several times and then use the method with which you feel the most comfortable and which does the best job for you.

Both meditation and relaxation are highly effective natural ways to handle stress. While both have the effect of getting you deeply calm and relaxed, the real benefits are in the rest of the day when this calm spreads into other phases of your activities. This calm state is the direct opposite of stress. Your breathing slows, your heartbeat is quiet, your metabolism lowers and your body recuperates during this period. The effects are gradual, but the more you practice, the greater they will be.

The meditation method is a way for you to let go of all the cares and worries that are on your mind. You release any thoughts you have other than the meditation. After making yourself comfortable in a chair, sofa or bed, loosen any tight clothing, close your eyes and relax. Focus your attention on your breath and its rhythm. If your mind wanders to any thought, bring it back to your breath. Just notice the easy and gentle passage of breath in and out of the nose. Don't try to control your breathing in any way. Just be aware of the situation. Be fully aware of the whole in-breath and the whole out-breath. This focus on your breath lets your body share the truly relaxed state. Some people like to say a comforting word of prayer with each breath like "health" or "peace." Some like to just be aware of each breath without saying anything. Stay awake. Do not allow yourself to fall asleep. Each meditation session is unique. There is no right way or wrong way to feel. Just keep track of your breathing and let happen whatever happens. Probably 10 to 15 minutes is long enough.

Our muscles store the tension of stress. To relax, we must first become aware of the difference between our tense state and that of deep relaxation. To use this second method, lie down on a thick carpet or mat, loosen any tight clothing, close your eyes and make yourself comfortable. Again, stay awake. The theory of this exercise is to tighten and relax each muscle. Begin by flexing your toes toward your knees. You will feel your calves tighten. Hold that tightly for 3 or 4 seconds and then let your toes relax and repeat. Lift your legs a few inches with your muscles tight, hold, drop them back and repeat. Tighten your buttocks hard, hold, relax, repeat. Hold your stomach way in, hold, relax, repeat. Take as deep a breath as possible, hold, exhale and repeat slowly. Relax as long as you feel comfortable between any of these exercises. Press your shoulders firmly to the floor arching your back, hold, release and repeat. Make your right hand into a tight fist, hold, relax and repeat. Bring your right hand to your right shoulder, make a muscle by tensing it, hold, relax and repeat. Repeat both of these with your left hand and arm. Shrug your shoulders toward your ears, hold, relax and repeat. Press your chin down against your chest, hold, relax and repeat. Close your eyes very tightly tensing your facial muscles, hold, relax and repeat. Clench your teeth tightening your jaw, hold, relax and repeat. Try to picture your whole body as soft and relaxed with a warmth spreading through every part. Imagine you have no more tension and your body is floating free. The sense of well-being, the healing sense, is filling your body and flowing through every part. Enjoy this deep relaxation for as long as you like.

Another method, the one I used most often, involves making yourself extremely comfortable in a chair, sofa or bed, loosening any tight clothing, closing your eyes and relaxing. Then, picture your forehead and say to yourself, "My forehead is relaxed." Then, picture your eyebrows and say, "My eyebrows are relaxed." Then your eyelids, your cheeks, your nose, your mouth, your chin and so forth down to your toes. By this time you should be fairly relaxed. Picture your body floating in an environment you particularly enjoy. I personally happen to like water, sunshine and trees. I pictured myself floating down a winding path beside a lake and finally lying in deep grass under tall trees with sunlight streaming through. You can use any other set of circumstances that you find appealing, comforting and relaxing.

Take this time for yourself to get calm, clear and deeply relaxed. A regular session of relaxation in and of itself is an antidote to the ravages of stress. Do this 3 times a day

– morning, mid-day and evening – for 15 to 20 minutes including your imagery. It has a cumulative effect that you will learn to enjoy and treasure.

While you are relaxed, realize that you are master of your body. It is yours to control, and it will care for you. It will follow your directions. A medical doctor wrote, "The greatest resource in medicine is within the patient himself."

Think about your thymus gland which is situated just under your breast bone. Direct your thymus gland to send out hundreds of thousands of new "T" cells that look like guard dogs, very protective of you. Send them to the parts of your body that you are the most concerned about. As you watch them go, whenever they find a cancer cell, they begin to eat and tear and devour those cancer cells. The cancer is fat, dumb and jelly-like. It cannot move, run or fight because it is a wrong cell that is not sup-posed to be there. It has no defense mechanism. Your "T" cells were designed specifically to search out and destroy these wrong cells. They are doing their job beautifully. Cancer cells are like raw hamburger: it is very easy for the "T" cells to completely eat them. They completely eradicate every cancer cell that is there. You can then picture that zone of your body clear and clean and free of cancer, pink and beautiful. Picture your "T" cells on a continuous search throughout your body detecting any cell that has gone wrong and killing it and flushing it from your system. You know these "T" cells are on guard 24 hours a day, protecting and defending you as they were designed to do.

Relax for a few moments. Stress reduces the function of the immune system and relaxation reduces stress. Each time you practice this, your relaxation should get deeper and more beneficial.

Another method of imagery is to picture your "T" cells as little shocks of electricity. They look like little lights streaming very vigorously out of your thymus gland. You watch them go to the part of the body with which you are most concerned, latch on to any cancer cells and shock and kill them. Some people prefer to picture their "T" cells as white knights in the form of "pac-man," a happy, aggressive white ball with only a mouth incessantly snapping, that searches out and devours all cancer cells.

No matter which of these methods you use, or one you might create, try it. Do it 3 times a day for 15 to 20 minutes each. Try different methods before you settle on one. Then use it for at least 10 consecutive days before thinking it is not for you. We are each supposed to learn something new every day. If this is your new knowledge for the day, you have done well for yourself, maybe helped to save your life.

For a graphic demonstration of what visual imagery is, create in your mind a vivid image of a ripe, yellow lemon squirting juice into your mouth and onto your tongue. You will actually begin to salivate. That is a clear example of how imagery can effect the nervous system, which regulates bodily processes and was traditionally thought to be beyond conscious control. If thinking of a juicy lemon makes you salivate, then what happens when you think of your life situation as hopeless? You are telling your immune system, "Don't bother! Don't do the best you can to heal me!" And to the contrary, when you image your medical treatments or your immune system as creating more mechanisms to kill your cancer, maybe that is just what it is doing.

There are no thorough studies yet that pinpoint the precise psychological mechanisms involved when emotions seem to affect health, says Leonard S. Zegans, M.D., professor of psychiatry at U.C.S.F. But, he adds, researchers believe that "hormones produced in response to emotional situations may affect lymphocytic (white blood cell) function and thus immunity to cancer, viral diseases and bacterial illnesses. Anything which gives a person a greater sense of control over the situation can be helpful. Information, for example, can relieve anxiety, and that can in turn improve a patient's chances for recovery."

Tapes to help you understand and practice relaxation are available from numerous sources including private practitioners and public libraries. If you have a problem finding one locally, you may borrow one free by sending a self-addressed, stamped envelope requesting "tape" to the Cancer Hot Line, 4400 Main, Kansas City, MO 64111.

Prayer 8

Prayer means many different things to different people. Before you jump to conclusions and believe you know everything about this subject as far as you are concerned, bear with me a minute. Maybe I picked the wrong word in choosing "prayer." Maybe it should have been emotional health, mental health or spiritual health. Probably best would be the term "spirituality." Every human being has spirituality. True spirituality is living what you believe. Spirituality denotes an interdependence which gets us out of loneliness. We are walking together. I've got my spiritual journey. You have yours. Maybe that is why you are reading this book, so that together maybe we can help you fight your cancer. Spiritualism is not what happened or why, but what you do with it and how you bear it.

When I was diagnosed with cancer, a friend gave me a subscription to *The Daily Word*. This is a small pamphlet that you receive in the mail each month with a page for each day of the month on which there is a prayer. I kept it next to my bed and first thing each morning I would read the prayer for that day. It made me feel very good. Often, at night, I felt like reading the prayer for the next day, but I would never "cheat." Some mornings I would wake up exceptionally early just to read the prayer. If you would like to subscribe to it for yourself or someone else, it is available from Unity School of Christianity, Unity Village, Missouri 64065.

M.D. Anderson, I was told when I went there, had an approximately 300-bed hospital with 6 full-time clergymen. It is one of the foremost scientific, research and treatment centers specializing in cancer in the country. This will indicate how they felt about prayer in the treatment of cancer. I know what it meant to me each day when a minister visited my room. It brightened my day and gave me a great lift, even though he was of a different faith.

Also, my section of the hospital had a sofa bed in each room on which the spouse of the patient could sleep. In the room next to mine was a foreign patient with his wife and 4 children living and cooking in his room. Again, this evidences M.D. Anderson's belief that cancer is a disease involving the entire family. Anything that can spiritually and mentally help the patient will contribute to their quality of life and recovery.

While I was recuperating from my surgery, a friend of mine who was studying for the ministry told me that since he had heard I was ill he had said a prayer for me every morning. You cannot possibly imagine what this simple statement meant to me. I told Annette that because of his prayers and those of others, I had no choice but to get well.

Each week I receive from the National Cancer Institute clippings run in papers around the country about cancer. One week I received an article that had nothing to do with cancer. That piqued my interest. It was about a double blind randomized trial run at the University of California-San Francisco, a very prestigious institution. It dealt with individuals admitted for open heart surgery. They were randomized by a computer into two groups, a trial group and a control group. Supposedly, these were identical because a patient with a good prognosis was placed in the trial group and the next patient with a good prognosis was placed in the control group. A patient with a poor prognosis was placed in the trial group and the next patient with a poor prognosis was placed in the control group.

The two groups were identical, and no one but the computer knew who was in which group. The doctors, the nurses and even the patients had no idea. The list of the trial group names was given to the students in a monastery who said prayers for the patients many times a day. They never met, and the patients never knew they were being prayed for. The files were unsealed some years later and reviewed and the results published because they were so startling. Those who were prayed for had a far faster recovery, far easier recovery with fewer side effects! Think of what the results might have been if the psychological aspects could have been added and they knew they were being prayed for!

What I'm trying to say here is to take a middle-of-the-road course. If you do, there is no possible way prayer can hurt you. If you are a logical, practical realist, there are only two possibilities. One: there is no God. If that would be true, it cannot hurt you to say a few prayers. Or two: there is a God watching over all of us. In that case it can help! Furthermore, it can stir up certain hormones within the body to help the immune system cure you.

My only comment to the religious fanatic, who believes he doesn't need medicine because God will take care of him, may sound facetious but is not meant that way. If God didn't want us to use medicine, why did he give us all these doctors? Why did he allow the scientists to develop all these revolutionary treatments? If a person believes that strongly in God, they must also believe that God helps those who help themselves. God intends for us to use all the wonderful things he has given us including doctors, nurses, hospitals and medicines.

A quote from a prayer book states, "Prayer cannot bring water to parched fields, or mend a broken bridge, or rebuild a ruined city; but prayer can water an arid soul, mend a broken heart, and rebuild a weakened will."

Bend In The Road
by Helen Steiner Rice

Sometimes we come to life's crossroads
And view what we think is the end.
But God has a much wider vision
And He knows that it's only a bend–
The road will go on and get smoother
And after we've stopped for a rest,
The path that lies hidden beyond us
Is often the path that is best.
So rest and relax and grow stronger,
Let go and let God share your load,
And have faith in a brighter tomorrow–
You've just come to a bend in the road.

Smoking 9

If you don't smoke or don't have cancer, you don't have to read this chapter. I have never tried to talk any person without cancer into quitting smoking. Everyone has read so much about it and knows how bad it is for their health and those around them that if they wanted to stop, they would. My criticizing them, trying to give them a guilty conscience or repeatedly suggesting they quit would do no good.

Tobacco has been proven beyond any reasonable doubt to be a carcinogen, a cancer causing agent. It was my understanding that any carcinogen was prohibited by federal law. However, because of the tobacco industry's powerful political lobby along with the clout of the owners of the cigarette vending machines, tobacco has been legislated exempt from all safety and health laws relating to carcinogens. Rather than try to convince millions of Americans to quit smoking, I believe it would be easier to convince 51% of the few hundred Congressmen and Senators to remove this exemption. I am not trying to put the tobacco companies out of business. I firmly believe that within 3 to 6 months they would be on the market with a product that could satisfy the need of people equally well without being a carcinogen. I have this much faith in American ingenuity. It can be done.

However, I was told where the fallacy lay in my reasoning. Cigarettes are blamed for 170,000 Americans' deaths each year from cancer. That's some 3,500 a week. These are the lives that could be saved from cancer. However, cigarettes kill some 500,000 Americans each year. Therefore, even if we could make them non-carcinogenic, they would still kill some 333,000 Americans from heart problems, lung problems and other causes. I nonetheless think it is worth saving the 170,000 Americans each year, and maybe the successor to the cigarette might not cause heart or lung problems.

Within seven seconds after a drag off a cigarette, the brain receives a "hit" of nicotine. The pack-and-a-half-per-day smoker will deliver about 350 drug hits of nicotine to the brain daily—that is 2,520 hits each week, 131,040 hits each year, or over seven million addictive hits in the smoker's lifetime. Not even eating is that successful a conditioned behavior!

Not all smokers, however, are nicotine dependent. There seems to be a spectrum with psychological dependence at one end and nicotine at the other. Possibly, individuals who successfully stop "cold turkey" on their own are at the psychological-dependence end while those who, like Mark Twain, have stopped hundreds of times "in the last year" are at the nicotine-dependent end of the spectrum.

A nicotine preparation impregnated in a gum complex is now available over the counter. If used properly, this nicotine gum should double long-term success rates in smoking cessation. To lower cardiac and pulmonary disease risk, to say nothing of cancer, the patient must stop smoking. There is no safe cigarette.

The reason I don't like to see a cancer patient smoking is much deeper than the fact that a cigarette is carcinogenic. I believe that for a person to overcome cancer, they must organize all their resources and do everything possible. They know that a cigarette is not good for them.

When I see a cancer patient light a cigarette, they are sending me a message. They might conquer cancer, but they are not willing to do everything possible to achieve that end result. They will beat it if it is convenient. I want to know that way deep down they are willing to do everything possible to beat cancer, and, if giving up smoking is part of the price they have to pay, then they will.

No one will say giving up smoking is fun or easy. I was a cigarette smoker for probably 35 years — some 2 to 2½ packs a day. Sure, I went to filters when they came out, and then I went to low tar and nicotine. I knew deep down that they were all bad for me. I justified it on the basis that I got so much pleasure from them and that my dad smoked all his life and didn't get cancer. When I finally quit, I found that I could enjoy life just as much or more without them. I sure paid the price for having smoked with my lung cancer.

How did I give them up? It wasn't easy, but this is why I never try to talk anyone else into quitting. I wanted to, and I believe that is the only way. I do not believe anyone can successfully give up smoking unless they really want to.

I woke up around 5 a.m. one morning in a hotel room with a beautiful view. I lay there looking out the open sliding doors. What a magnificent sight, I thought to myself. I think I want to stick around and watch this for a while. I am not going to smoke today. I don't know about tomorrow, but I am not going to smoke today. I remembered hearing about the methods of Alcoholics Anonymous where they never give up drinking but just don't drink from one day to the next. Well, this is what I've been doing with cigarettes for many years now. It is possible that I could smoke tomorrow, but I know I won't smoke today.

Sure, it was tough, but what rewards I have reaped. First, I realized my life is every bit as pleasant and even more so than before. I don't worry about dropping ashes and burning tables, clothes or whatever. I don't have that bad taste in my mouth, bad breath or stains on my fingers and teeth. Food tastes good. I'm not hoarse, and I lost the persistent cough. Most of all, I would have hated to have to give up cigarettes simultaneously with the treatments I went through, or any other medical treatments for that matter.

When my doctor was going to give me chemotherapy, it was suggested that I smoke marijuana to reduce the possible nausea. I refused because I know the anguish I went through in stopping, and I would rather be nauseated than go through quitting again. No one has to tell me how tough it is to quit.

It's no fun, but it can be done. If you really want to live and beat cancer, you will do everything in your power to accomplish this. You know smoking cannot help you. It can only hurt you. It is one of the things you have in your power to do something about. If you are honest and you sincerely want to try to beat cancer, prove it by not taking another cigarette today.

Pain Relief 10

"My own feeling is that no cancer patient today should have to suffer severely from physical pain," states Dr. Vincent T. DeVita, Jr., former director of the National Cancer Institute. "First of all, only 20 to 30 percent of cancer patients get severe pain; the rest don't. For those patients who have pain, there are plenty of drugs on the market to cover almost every kind of pain. We also have neurosurgical procedures to relieve pain. The main problem is that doctors are not taught how to use narcotics in medical school, and they usually don't prescribe painkillers frequently enough. The fear that some patients may become addicted to narcotics is frankly ludicrous in patients who are dying of cancer. No patient should have to ask for pain relief."

Cancer patients may like to take a pain relieving drug because they feel comfortable when they do. This is not addiction. It is a very rare happening, really most unusual for a cancer patient to become addicted because of drugs taken while they have cancer.

Take medicine according to your doctor's advice. Don't be concerned with addiction. Often, a smaller amount of medication before feeling pain can avoid having to take a much larger dose later to ease the pain.

As a cancer patient, you may get infuriated when you hear the discussion as to why Congress will not legalize the use of heroin for cancer patients. Before you fly off the handle, give some thought as to why the American Medical Association, the American Society of Internal Medicine and the Medical Society of the State of New York among others are opposed to legalizing the use of heroin. It is because heroin is not the only solution to the problem of intractable pain. A drug that many pharmaceutical and medical experts consider more effective than heroin is Dilaudid, which is legal and has been available for some time. It is highly soluble, more potent, achieves its peak effect sooner and has a longer duration of action than heroin.

Our bodies are built to send messages to the brain when something is wrong. Pain is just such a message. Possibly, it helped you in finding an earlier diagnosis. Often, by improving the quality of life, by doing things we enjoy, by having pleasure and forgetting our cares and problems, we can diminish our pain. This does not mean our pain is imaginary. It only means that we have the power to replace it with something positive.

Norman Cousins found that watching funny movies had an excellent effect on him, making him forget his pain. There is an old saying, "Laughter is the best medicine." Several hospitals have put in a "laughing room" where tapes of funny movies are continuously shown for the benefit of cancer patients. Others are talking of dedicating one channel of their closed circuit television to this same type of programming. We're not all the same, but for many of us, it can have a very beneficial effect.

When side effects of treatments are particularly severe, it could be because you feel out of control and are resisting your doctor's treatments. If you can get back to feeling in control, if you participate with your doctor in deciding on the treatment, if you want the treatment, if you believe the treatment will help you, if you practice visualization during the treatment, often the side effects will be diminished. We can bear much more discomfort when we believe the results will be worthwhile.

Acute pain can depress a patient and reduce the will to live. The important thing is to get the pain stopped. Don't cry wolf for every little ache and pain, but when it gets serious, let your doctor know and be certain he gets rid of it.

There are many recognized ways to treat pain in addition to drugs. These would include psychological therapy of an individual or group nature, biofeedback, hypnosis, physical therapy and massage. Furthermore, it is not necessary to concentrate all your hopes on one specific method. Generally, it is possible to resort to several methods simultaneously. Some believe that the more kinds of treatment you receive, the more your pain will decrease, in that each treatment can have not only a cumulative but a synergistic effect on the others.

Radiation is recognized as one definite way to eliminate or dramatically reduce pain in many situations. These treatments are known as palliative treatments in that they are strictly to make the patient feel better by killing the cancer in a local area but generally will not cure the overall disease. Certain chemotherapies are used to make the patient feel better. These are but two examples of where the treatments that have such a bad reputation in fact are given for the exact opposite reason, to make the patient feel better. Check with your physician to see if it is appropriate for you.

When I was taking chemotherapy, the extremely potent drugs were making me very sick, weak and thoroughly miserable. True, life in that state was absolutely not worthwhile. I was not only in physical pain, but mental and emotional pain as well. However, realizing that if those drugs were making this great big body of mine that sick and weak, they were also playing havoc with those weak, dumb cancer cells and destroying them. These horrible drugs were giving me a chance to live. Not only did my positive thinking enable me to tolerate the pain, I actually looked forward to being made sick because I knew it was giving me a chance to live. Always remember that the purpose of cancer treatments is to help you. Welcome them, understand them, help them to do their job and be grateful to the doctors and scientists who discovered them, perfected them and are giving them to you.

I had never been a pill taker. My surgeon insisted that I take a pain killer every four hours after surgery. That was five pills a day, each containing one grain of codeine. He explained that the surgery had left a great deal of scar tissue in my shoulder. A little pain medication taken regularly, before pain and the resulting tension started, would keep me relatively free of pain and allow me to heal faster.

Again, I am not a pill taker. Twice–once in July on our way to Bermuda and a second time in August at home–I tried to break the habit. Both times, on the second day, the pain was intolerable, and I had to go back to using the codeine.

On my next regular visit to Houston, the doctor recommended that I see the M.D. Anderson staff psychologist. We visited him the afternoon we were leaving. I explained that I did not believe in psychiatrists or psychologists. I felt that I was an intelligent individual and was able to control my thoughts without help.

He started off by saying that since I was leaving that afternoon, he would be unable to treat me, so he would like to tell me a story. Subconsciously, this established my confidence in him, since he could have no personal motive.

He told me to picture myself walking across Main Street with a tremendously sore leg. Each step means excruciating pain. I am barely able to hop. In the middle of Main Street, I glance up and suddenly see a huge truck coming at me at 60 mph. What happens? Suddenly, I have no pain, and I am easily able to run the rest of the way across the street to avoid being hit by the truck. When I reach the curb and stop, the pain is back in full force. What does this prove? The mind is capable of turning off pain if it wants to.

He recommended that when we got home, we find a psychologist who specializes in pain. My wife made numerous phone calls and did a great deal of research before finally making an appointment with a doctor. He explained that pain was a combination of two factors: tension and physical hurt. If I could learn to relax and get rid of tension, the pain would be less severe. I always thought of myself as a very relaxed person, but I did not know the true meaning of the word.

On the first visit, he taught me to relax by the third method described in chapter 5. I was to do this every morning and evening. I was really relaxed.

On my second visit a week later, after relaxing me, the doctor attempted to use hypnosis to stop the pain. It did not work. A week later on the third visit, he tried again without success.

On the fourth week, after relaxing me, he asked me to think of the most beautiful thought in the world and tell him what it was. I said it was my wife's love for me. He then said that my body was filling with my wife's love for me and repeated that it was completely filling my entire body. I took my good left hand and placed it on the left side of my chest and rubbed it across to my right shoulder forcing my wife's love for me into the right shoulder and all the pain out. It worked. From the time I left the doctor's office that day, I never took another pain pill. Whenever my shoulder started hurting, I thought of my wife's love for me and forced it up into my shoulder and instantly the pain was gone.

This story was not for the purpose of entertaining or impressing you. It is meant to emphasize four critical points.

First, take any pain medications in accordance with your doctor's recommendations.

Second, stress and tension do play a dramatic part in the feeling of pain.

Third, if something doesn't work the first time, don't give up. If it is good and has worked for others, keep on trying. We are all individuals, and everything will not work for each one of us, but there is probably a variation that will help.

Fourth, in pain as in everything else, seek a qualified professional who specializes strictly in that field. He knows current state-of-the-art therapy off the top of his head along with all possible options.

Diet 11

Diet is an extremely critical part of the successful treatment of cancer. However, a couple words of caution before you go off the deep end. Don't confuse the recommended diet for avoiding cancer with the recommendations for helping cure cancer. There is absolutely no relationship. Books have been written on diet to prevent cancer. That is not what we are concerned with here. You have cancer, and you want to recover.

The critical part of diet is to eat a well-balanced diet to help maintain your strength so that your own body is capable of aiding the medical treatments in doing their job. Your immune system, to a degree, is dependent on proper nourishment. Every professional I have talked with speaks in terms of calories, vitamins and minerals, always in moderation and well balanced but sufficient to support your body even though you may not feel like it.

Often, patients lose their appetite due to the treatments or to the disease itself. In this case, it is important, even critical, to force yourself to eat a sufficient and well-balanced diet to give your system proper nourishment. This is no time to even think about dieting. Try your best to maintain your weight.

Of course, all of this must be tailored to the patient's needs by their personal physician. For patients who are losing excessive weight, a high fat diet may be recommended. For those whose treatments make it difficult or impossible to eat, health professionals will encourage any intake of food which provides calories, even if that means a diet of ice cream sodas.

The second word of caution is to look carefully at any purported cure that is based on a specific diet. Where, other than psychologically, is the potential benefit? I have looked in depth into such fad cures as macrobiotics, megadoses of certain vitamins, coffee enemas and even Laetrile. They are appealing to an individual who has been denied hope by a physician or a person who does not want to work within the medical system and is looking for the easy way. Believe me, if it were there, it would be well documented. There would be many more successes than those who were cured by spontaneous remission or psychotherapy. Don't get me wrong. Spontaneous remission and psychotherapy are wonderful, but they can be more often successful, in my opinion, when applied with orthodox medical treatments than alternative therapies.

Researchers believe that the mechanisms at work in response to hopefulness are identical to those involved with placebos. If you believe that a treatment for an ailment will be helpful, you are much more likely to benefit from it. The placebo effect has often been used to explain why treatments like Laetrile seem to cure some cancer patients even though credible scientific studies have never found therapeutic value in such treatments.

The Food and Nutrition Board of the National Research Council, in a publication entitled *Toward Healthful Diets*, stated, "Sound nutrition is not a panacea. Good food that provides appropriate proportions of nutrients should not be regarded as a poison, a medicine, or a talisman. It should be eaten and enjoyed." What upset many was the board's conclusion that there was no specific dietary advice appropriate for all. The board recommended balance in food selection tempered with moderation in consumption.

Many people today have unrealistic notions about what nutrition can accomplish. Certain enthusiasts even claim nutrition can cure cancer.

Nutrition does play an important role in the prevention and treatment of cancer, but it is not a cure-all. This view is supported by Dr. Richard Rivlin, chief of nutrition services at the Memorial Sloan-Kettering Cancer Center in New York. "It is a tragedy when nutrition is viewed as the sole means of prevention and treatment of cancer, particularly when established methods of attacking the disease by surgery, radiotherapy or chemotherapy are abandoned for the illusory benefits of a 'holistic approach' using nutrition exclusively," said Dr. Rivlin.

He added, "Nutrition is an important adjunct to any treatment plan, one that has often not been utilized enough, but nutrition should not be expected to do the job entirely on its own."

Nutrition is essential while a patient receives drug and radiation therapy. One technique, called hyper-alimentation, involves intravenous feeding with a concentrated solution of nutrients that enable the patient to maintain weight without eating. This keeps a patient strong enough to fight the disease.

Careful scientific studies have shown that "organic" diets, coffee enemas, megadoses of certain vitamins, and the use of Laetrile or pangamic acid are of no value in the treatment of cancer. As a matter of fact, megadoses of certain vitamins such as A, D, E and K can be damaging. Laetrile, in particular, is harmful because its cyanide content can be quite toxic.

While vitamin C has been demonstrated in controlled tests to have no benefit in fighting cancer, many people ask about it. Possibly, this is because Linus Pauling, who won a Nobel Prize in a completely unrelated field, recommends it highly. My advice to you is to talk to your physician. Under certain circumstances, it could counteract the beneficial effects of a particular cancer drug. If your doctor says it will not hurt you, take it if you personally believe in its merits.

On a visit to Fox Chase Cancer Center, I was discussing with Dr. Sears, an oncologic surgeon interested in immunology, successes he was having with an experimental protocol using monoclonal antibodies. He stated that one patient came for a check-up with extremely yellow skin. Dr. Sears asked the patient how he was feeling and he replied that he felt perfect. He volunteered that if the doctor was worrying about the color of his skin, it was because he was taking 50,000 units of carotene a day!

Dr. Sears told me that there were three patients on this protocol who were doing outstandingly well. He had realized that each of these three were taking megadoses of something, each different, because they believed in it, and he had assured them it would not conflict with their treatment.

I have thought about these comments and come to certain conclusions. First, since each of the substances were different, it was obviously not the substance that benefited the patient. Three out of three is such a small number that it could have been strictly chance that each who did so well took a megadose of something.

I prefer to believe that the result is a combination of two more likely scenarios. First, is that of a placebo. The patient, believing the megadose would help, actually aided the monoclonal antibodies or their own immune system in destroying the cancer. Even more important, I believe, is the fact that this demonstrates that these people are fighters. They are not willing to sit back and do nothing. They were not even willing to sit back and let their doctor try to treat them with a great new treatment. They were going to do everything in their power to fight this disease. Maybe, and I think this is most likely, this demonstration of dedication and determination gave them the infinitesimal advantage to tip the scales in their favor and make the combination of everything actually accomplish the purpose for which it was intended.

Nutrition is an important consideration to every cancer patient; however, it provides the best results only when approached with realistic expectations. Eat a well-balanced diet sufficient to maintain your strength and follow your qualified physician's advice.

Conclusions 12

What you have read in this book is probably different from anything you have ever believed about your body and its functions. My hope is that, on some level at least, parts of it make some sense to you. I can assure you everything in this book has been suggested by some test or research somewhere. See if you can't say to yourself that you are willing to try each suggestion, if for no other reason than you don't see how it can do any harm. Then try, try the whole thing by trying every little detail. Only after you have tried something, do you have the right to say with authority that it is not for you.

Sometimes 2 plus 2 equals 5 or 6 or 7. Take a tiny acorn, some dirt, water and sunshine. Each of these is an innocuous little thing on its own, but add them all together

LIVES ARE NOT LOST TO CANCER—
THEY ARE *PILFERED*
BY THE VICTIMS THEMSELVES!

Procrastination: I'm feeling too good and I'm too busy. I'll get it treated when I have more time (not realizing that cancer grows geometrically).

Ignorance: There are at least 6 common, separate methods to treat cancer. Death and cancer are not synonymous.

Laziness: When the doctor who discovers it says to wait and see or that there is nothing that can be done, the easy way out is to accept that statement.

Fear: Of the horrible treatments because you heard how someone suffered years ago to no avail. We've come a long way baby.

Expectation or desire to die: If you do, you will.

Reliance: On a general doctor's opinion without seeking the thoroughness, expertise and accuracy of a second opinion by a board certified oncologist, a doctor qualified to treat cancer and specializing in treating cancer.

and give them some time and you have a magnificent, gigantic oak tree.

Maybe some ideas don't work too well on their own, but when done in conjunction with something else, you have a winner. And isn't that what it is all about — having a winner? Does it really make that much difference how you get there? If you do everything and you get well, then and only then can you afford the luxury of looking back and trying to decide which factors were influential in your recovery.

This book would not be complete without at least a mention of luck. It is one of the five factors to which I attribute my cure. The fact that my tumor formed around a nerve in my shoulder and hurt so much, forcing me back to physicians repeatedly, in spite of assurances that it was not cancer, was luck, pure and simple. Of course, I could look at the negative side of things and say that finding the first two doctors who wrongly diagnosed it was "bad luck" because it stole precious time. What would that get me? It would make me nervous and upset, wasting valuable energy thinking negative thoughts.

Concentrate on the positive and get on in your fight against cancer.

If the grass is greener on the other side of the street, is that truly luck? Or did our neighbor do all those little things that we thought were too unpleasant or didn't matter that much. The harder you work, the luckier you get. If you want to have good luck in getting rid of your cancer, apply yourself and work for it. Nothing worthwhile comes easily.

A young woman called, telling me her mother was dying of cancer, refusing all medical treatments and even denying that she had cancer. Her father would not discuss it with anyone. But this young woman said she knew her mother would make it because she believed a miracle would happen. It was my opinion that miracles or luck don't just happen, you have to make them happen. It is hard work that will give her mother a chance. She must find competent psychological assistance to convince her mother of the problem and to do everything in her power to overcome it, and then maybe a miracle is possible.

The purpose of this is not to instill guilt in anyone. Everyone cannot beat cancer, no matter how hard they try. In trying to bring about your own luck, you are kept busy working which, in itself, provides you a better quality of life, and maybe you can succeed.

Harold Benjamin, founder of the Wellness Community, stated in the *Los Angeles Times*, "Listen, when I first started the Wellness group, everybody said, 'Don't give them false hope,' and for a while I really gave that some credence. But you know what? There's no such thing as false hope. If we told them, 'If you do certain things, you'll get better, guaranteed,' that would be either stupidity or fraud. But if 1 out of 500 people get well, is it unreasonable to hope you'll be that one person? Not to me it isn't."

"Hope is an essential part of the will to live," states Dr. Ernest Rosenbaum in his book, *Living with Cancer*. "Hope can be maintained as long as there is even a remote chance for survival. It is kindled and nurtured by even minor improvements and is maintained when crises or reversals persist by the positive attitudes of family, friends, and the health support team. Primarily, though, hope will come from within you, if you are willing to do everything you can do to improve your health and if you are willing to fight for your life."

Dr. Lewis Thomas, former chancellor of Memorial Sloan-Kettering, said, "From time to time patients turn up with advanced cancer, beyond possibility of cure...The patient is sent home to die, only to turn up again ten years later free of disease and in good health. There are now several hundred such cases in world scientific literature, and no one doubts the validity of the observations."

At the dedication of the R.A. Bloch International Cancer Information Center in Bethesda, MD, I declared, "Having been told I was terminal from lung cancer and subsequently cured by top physicians, I as much as anyone appreciate the fact that it is doctors and knowledge that cure cancer, not bricks and mortar. Over one half of the cases of cancer that were untreatable when a young doctor completed medical school only 20 years ago are today curable to some degree.

Tremendous strides are being made continuously in the treatment of various types of cancer. It is obvious that some people are dying, not because there is no treatment for their cancer, but because their doctor is unaware of the latest and best treatments. It is Annette's and my hope that this building will be the catalyst to disseminating state-of-the-art information to the physicians of the world to enable them to improve the quality and quantity of life for every cancer patient."

Being told you have cancer is like being hit by a truck. In a few seconds, the course of your life is altered. Shock! Fear! Guilt! Anger! Bewilderment! These are reactions of many cancer patients when told they have cancer. You should do everything possible to maximize your chances of beating cancer. The following are a few suggestions:

1. The fact that you have cancer cannot be changed. Right now is the most important time in decision-making—at the very beginning— when numerous alternatives may be open to you.

2. As a cancer patient, you must be an activist. You must become a partner with your doctor. Understand everything that is being suggested and why. Ask questions. Educate yourself on your specific type of cancer. Get all the information you can from the Cancer Information Service and visit a medical library. So much successful research is being accomplished daily that you may find a clue to a potential treatment.

3. Demand to know all the alternatives. If you make a decision to go ahead with a treatment without sufficient testing or a qualified second opinion, you may be limiting the possibility of other therapies right from the start. Often, unless you remain calm and in control, a decision is made for you by circumstances that will take it out of your control. Learning all you can about your case and the alternatives means you can control the way your illness is handled.

4. For all serious cancers, a second opinion from a board certified oncologist is an absolute must before submitting to any treatment of any kind. Requesting a second opinion does not mean the diagnosis you were given is not correct or that the suggested treatment is not the best. It is only to say that you deserve the right to have the doctor's diagnosis confirmed and optional treatments explored and explained to you. At least, it will afford you peace of mind in knowing that everything your original doctor told you is correct.

5. Death and cancer are no longer synonymous. Most people can be successfully treated by established medical treatments. Ignore unproven "easy" methods which promise cures by people who purport to be suppressed by the medical profession. Rely on established medical treatments plus supplemental suggestions as outlined in this book and stay far away from alternative therapies in lieu of orthodox medicine.

6. Most people want to know their odds of cure. Remember, you are not a statistic, you are a single human being. You may have better family support; you may have better medical attention; you may have a stronger desire to live; you may have a more positive outlook; you may be willing to become more involved, etc., etc. etc. Statistics can be fun to play with, but they are no more than averages. If you recover, your chances are 100%. If you don't, they are zero. There is no type of cancer from which some people have not recovered. Make up your mind that you are going to do everything in your power to be one of these and forget about the rest.

7. You, as a cancer patient, are a consumer. As a consumer, you have the right to ask questions and to expect answers in terms you can understand. Doctors often seem so busy that a patient feels guilty and apologetic for taking up their time. Keep a running list of questions for your doctor and go over each one with him. By taking an active interest in your case, you will be showing your doctor you have joined him in the fight against your cancer.

8. Always have a family member or friend with you when discussing your case with your doctor. This reduces the possibility of misunderstanding and eliminates the need for repetition. There is also the therapeutic value of treating the family as a unit.

9. Be certain you differentiate between the possible and probable side effects of your proposed treatment. Your doctors must explain all the possible side effects to you, but request that the probable effects be enumerated. You will find that of the many possible things that could happen, very few actually should happen. Also, some patients mistakenly interpret these side effects as their cancer worsening, when in reality they are the normal effects of their treatments and their cancer is probably getting better.

10. Expect some degree of depression. Cancer is a serious illness. Many of the treatments are depressants. "Down days" will occur from time to time. Plan on ways of coping with them. Call a friend. Take a walk. Do something you really enjoy.

11. Throughout your cancer treatment, maintain as normal a life as possible. Set goals and have someone or something to live for. You will feel much better about yourself, and it will help you cope with your treatment.

Not minimizing the pain, stress and fear that accompany cancer and its treatment, it is a fact that everything does not necessarily have to be negative. It is possible that through this illness you can learn to live a better and fuller life.

Q. I've heard a great deal of discussion about certain diets curing cancer. What can you tell me about this or vitamins to cure my cancer?

A. The discussion of vitamins and diet must be separated into two distinct categories: causing cancer and curing cancer. Because of your question, my answer will be limited to their effect on cures.

The four most important factors in the successful treatment of cancer are prompt treatment, proper treatment, thorough medical treatment and a positive mental attitude. This is the tried and proven way which in my opinion would lead to the successful treatment of more serious cancers today. Anything in lieu of orthodox therapies is looking for the easy way out and could lead to disaster. I have done a great deal of reading and been exposed to much discussion on diet curing cancer through my position on the National Cancer Advisory Board. What I have gathered from the leading scientists is that it is critical for cancer patients to eat a well-balanced diet and attempt to maintain their weight and energy during debilitating treatments. This will allow their bodies to help fight the cancer along with the treatments.

To date, no specific diets or vitamins have been proved statistically to have any curative powers. Therefore, if you believe that a particular diet or vitamin would aid in the successful treatment of your cancer, ask your doctor. If he says it will not hurt you, do it along with the recommended medical treatments. This can create a positive mental attitude, which is a critical thing in beating cancer when used in addition to, not in lieu of, medical treatment.

Q. There are so many things I don't understand about my cancer, and yet I am afraid to ask my doctor too many foolish questions.

A. The only bad question is the one you didn't ask! So many times people are afraid to ask questions. They fear they may sound silly or offend their doctor. In reality, their doctor would like them to ask any question on their mind. The doctor cannot guess what the patient wants to know.

Any qualified oncologist I have talked to agrees that treatment will have a better chance of success if the patient understands the what, why and how of it. If you do not understand your doctor's explanation, keep questioning until you are satisfied in your mind that you do understand. Your physician will appreciate it. Keep a blank sheet of paper in a convenient place and, every time a question comes to mind, write it down. This way you will not fail to ask something that has been bothering you. You will have a better chance of beating cancer if you will allow your doctor to treat the patient, not just the disease, and this includes you understanding everything about your illness and your treatments.

Q. On a routine annual physical, my doctor discovered I had a malignancy. He wants me to promptly start with treatments that could be debilitating. Since I feel so well and it's the busiest time of the year for me, what harm would it be to put the treatments off for a few months?

A. First of all, be very grateful that your doctor discovered your cancer when he did. The earlier you catch cancer, generally the better the prognosis. Since you're feeling so good, the chances are you found it very early.

Remember that cancer grows geometrically. Cancer is never as treatable as it is today. All treatments are easier or work better on small amounts of malignant cells.

Supposedly, everyone gets cancer six times a year. While there is some doubt, it has been suggested that the immune system is capable of killing these few malignant cells, and the person stays healthy. It is only when these cells multiply to a point where the immune system cannot destroy them that you have a detectable cancer. When you allow this to multiply to some point, it becomes totally untreatable.

Be grateful your malignancy was discovered early. Follow your doctor's advice. Get your cancer behind you so you can live a long, healthy life and enjoy many busy seasons in the future.

Q. I was just told I had cancer. Would you recommend I go out of town for treatment?

A. It is doctors and knowledge that cure cancer, not bricks and mortar. Cancer that is treated promptly, properly and thoroughly has an excellent chance of recovery if you have a positive mental attitude.

If your cancer is an extremely rare type for which highly experimental therapy is being given on a very restricted basis, I would go where this experimental therapy is being given. If you must be treated with equipment not locally available, such as hyperthermia for ovarian cancer, I would go where it is available. Otherwise, you will generally find doctors in your community as qualified as those anywhere. There are numerous large, cooperative groups that share protocols. These can be obtained locally as well as at a major center.

I worry about your frame of mind, since you ask the question. Assuming the physician you are going to is qualified to treat cancer, I urge you to ask him if you should go out of town or get a second opinion. There is no doubt you will receive an honest answer that will allow you to have total peace of mind, a necessary ingredient in the successful treatment of cancer.

Q. What is the connection between mental attitude and the incidence of cancer?

A. While there is some debate over this, it is interesting to note that scientists have proven that mice under stress get cancer at a greater rate than mice allowed to live peacefully. Also, tumors grow faster in mice under stress. A leading psychiatrist found a higher incidence of cancer in people with suicidal tendencies. It is known that the incidence of cancer goes up after the death of a parent, spouse or child, divorce, retirement, bankruptcy, etc. Personally, I don't recall talking with a cancer patient who did not have a traumatic event in their life six months to three years prior to their cancer.

When people ask me what to do to keep them from getting cancer, I first suggest not smoking, because that is the biggest single known cause of cancer. Eat a proper, well-balanced diet, learn to cope with the stress in your life as well as possible, don't worry and think positive. Remember, three out of four people don't get cancer. Make up your mind you're one of the three out of four; and if you're wrong, you still have at least a 50 percent chance of beating it. In other words, don't worry and live a good, healthy life.

Q. What is the connection between mental attitude and the successful treatment of cancer?

A. The subject is scientifically unproved. I have never met an oncologist who did not agree that people with cancer who believe they will die from it compromise their chances of survival. Even with the simplest, most treatable cancer, there is often no way to successfully treat someone who wants to die or thinks he will die. However, some patients can be cured in spite of themselves. One psychiatrist called cancer a legal method of committing suicide. That is not to say that, if you think you will get well, you will, but at least then you have a chance.

There is a saying, "Nice guys don't win the fight against cancer." Meek, mild-mannered people who are afraid to question their doctors, who don't understand or get involved, tend not to do as well.

In my opinion, a system of complete mental relaxation along with having an image of your cancer and thinking it away could be helpful. It is recommended, like prayer, in addition to any medical treatments by your doctor. I used it when I was being treated. I personally believe it helped. I know it improved the quality of my life, and I am positive it did not hurt me.

Cancer is a very serious disease. There is generally only one chance to beat it. Muster all your resources and do everything possible the first time, so you will never look back and be sorry. Include relaxation, imagery and a positive mental attitude, because they can only help and cannot hurt.

Q. As a result of my cancer, the linings of my nerves were destroyed to a point where I cannot use my arms or legs. My doctor believes they can cure my cancer but gives me no more than a 5 percent chance of getting the use of my arms and legs back. Is it worth going through the ordeal of treatment with those odds?

A. Let's go one step at a time. You have two choices: to try to fight your cancer and live, or to give up, in which case you will die. You are fortunate, because some individuals with cancer cannot be treated. If you try to fight it, the quality of your life will be greatly improved, even if the quantity or physical agility will not. If you are successful in beating your cancer, maybe you will be successful in beating your disability.

You are a human being, not a statistic! Who knows? Maybe you will be that one out of 20 to overcome your problem. Tremendous strides are being made in medical treatment. We don't know what will be discovered this afternoon or tomorrow. If you're not alive, it can't do you any good.

After my cancer surgery, my doctor told me that I would never play tennis again because he had to remove a major nerve in my right arm. I lost total use of my arm until I made up my mind I was going to do something about it. After an extended period of intense physical therapy, including shock treatments, I am now playing tennis better than ever.

If you don't try, you can't succeed. I'm not saying you can make it if you try, but at least you have a chance.

Q. As a former cancer patient, how much do you think a patient should be told about his condition?

A. In the days when cancer was synonymous with death, many patients were intentionally not told they had cancer. Recently, I have never talked with an oncologist who believed in anything other than complete truth and honesty.

Complete truth and honesty would include the gravity of the situation as well as the options and prognosis. Where there is life, there is hope.

John Porter, a former president of our Cancer Hot Line, has said that a human being could live for 30 days without food, could exist for seven days without water and could last four minutes without air, but a human being could not exist for 10 seconds without hope.

This is not to be confused with false hope, although Dr. Vincent T. DeVita Jr., former director of the National Cancer Institute, says that there is no type of cancer from which some people have not recovered.

If a patient is told the statistics of his disease, he should be reminded that he is a human being and not a statistic. He may have a stronger desire to live and greater support from family and friends, may have better medical attention, may have caught the problem earlier or be in better physical condition than the average patient, so statistics do not apply to him. If he makes it, his chances are 100 percent; if he doesn't, his chances are zero.

I personally am in favor of the patient knowing everything about their disease. This way they can participate in and become a part of their treatment, improve the quality of their life and aid the chance of a favorable outcome.

Q. What is meant by a multidisciplinary opinion?

A. Because cancer is more than 100 different diseases and there are at least six primary forms of cancer treatment, it is impossible for any single doctor to know the latest and best treatment for every type of cancer. A doctor who knew the latest surgical technique for a specific type of cancer could be unaware of the up-to-the-minute chemotherapy, immunization therapy, hyperthermia or radiation therapy for that particular type of cancer.

A multidisciplinary opinion means getting together physicians from various specialties (disciplines), depending on the type of cancer, such as a pathologist, a diagnostic radiologist, a medical oncologist, a surgeon and a radiation oncologist. They discuss the type of cancer, the location, the stage, all the possible treatments and then recommend, in order, the preferred series of treatments most likely to successfully treat that particular patient.

Remember that many cancers can be successfully treated if they are treated promptly, properly and thoroughly. To ensure that you are doing everything you possibly can to help yourself beat this insidious disease, I would strongly recommend getting a multidisciplinary opinion before any treatment, if at all possible.

Q. I am feeling wonderful. I have just finished a series of radiation treatments which my doctor says may have cured my cancer. However, he wants me to keep taking adjuvant chemotherapy to be on the safe side. Since I'm feeling good, shouldn't I wait until there's a recurrence before going through the ordeal of chemotherapy?

A. Adjuvant chemotherapy is given when there is no actual physical evidence that cancer exists but it is likely to be present in the body in minute quantities.

One million cancer cells are smaller than the head of a pin. Chemotherapy is most effective against small quantities of cancer and could be totally ineffective against large masses.

After I had radiation, chemotherapy and immunotherapy for my lung cancer, the surgery showed no living cancer cells. My doctor wanted me to take one more year of chemotherapy. He explained the chances were 95 percent I didn't need it. If I did get a recurrence, however, I would be dead.

I had five friends with similar lung cancers who were all told they were "cured" after surgery and that chemotherapy was not necessary. The doctor and my wife gave me no choice but to take the chemotherapy. My five friends are all dead from their cancers.

Be grateful that they discovered the drugs and that you have such a thorough doctor. Cancer is one disease for which no one can afford the luxury of looking back and saying, "I wish I would have..."

Q. My doctor just told me that I have to take chemotherapy to recover from cancer. I have heard so many horror stories about it, such as getting violently ill and losing your hair. Is it worth it?

A. Chemotherapy is treating the body with chemicals. Taking two aspirin is chemotherapy. Cancer chemotherapy covers a spectrum. Many drugs create absolutely no side effects such as those you describe. On the other hand, a drug called Adriamycin is affectionately known as "the Red Devil" because of the side effects it may cause. Most people have never heard of it, but Adriamycin saves more lives every year from cancer than the Salk vaccine saves from polio.

Sure, some drugs are rough to take, but the idea is not to take treatments. The idea is to get rid of the cancer. I knew that if these drugs were making this big body of mine so sick and so infirm, they were absolutely destroying those little cancer cells. I dreaded the miserable feeling of nausea each month, but I actually looked forward to being made sick because I knew it gave me a chance to live.

Today, chemotherapy, like radiation, is a science. It is not witchcraft. It is not guesswork. Your qualified oncologist knows exactly how much of a particular drug must be administered to destroy tumor cells and do no damage to any organ.

In answer to your question, be grateful that scientists and doctors discovered and perfected these drugs so that you have a chance to live. Having been there, it is my feeling that seeing the sun come up one more morning is worth every treatment I went through.

Q. I feel very uncomfortable discussing my cancer because I don't want to be pitied. My husband says I am wrong. Who is right?

A. Your feeling of not wanting sympathy is understandable. At a time like this, however, it's most important to have the support of your family and friends. The normal worry and fear from the shock of finding you have cancer and the impending treatments is a tremendous burden to carry alone. Share your feelings with your family and friends. Not only will it help you, but it will make them feel more comfortable. They want to be helpful to you, but they can't if you shut them out. Talk about it openly, not incessantly.

Cancer is not a dirty word or something to be ashamed of, nor is it something to brag about or discuss continuously. Act your normal self and follow your doctor's advice with help from those who care about you.

Q. I have heard of a computer program about cancer in which you are somehow involved. Can you tell me something about it?

A. The program you are referring to is called PDQ by the National Cancer Institute and is housed in the R.A. Bloch International Cancer Information Center in Bethesda, MD. I spent many sleepless nights formulating the plans for this program.

After I was cured, I realized others were dying, not because they could not be cured, but because cancer is such a complex disease and their physicians were not aware of the recent developments. Billions of dollars have been spent. Thousands of scientists and doctors spend their lives developing treatments, but if the one doctor treating the patient is unaware of the state-of-the-art therapy for that particular cancer, everything is wasted.

The idea was to get every treatment for every type of cancer from every center in the country into a computer. Then a doctor anywhere could call this computer with his computer, explain the type of cancer and immediately he would be advised of all the options. The National Cancer Institute has gone a step or two further by getting more than 22 countries to list their protocols in the system, and they give a state-of-the-art statement for each known cancer.

This has been a monumental task that could never have been done by any other organization. The National Cancer Institute and its employees have done an incredibly outstanding job. This program is available to any physician or patient simply by calling 1-800-4-CANCER and specifically requesting PDQ for a particular type and stage of cancer including the state-of-the-art therapy and all current open protocols on a national basis in short form. It is also available instantly by computer from the National Library of Medicine and various private sources.

The exciting thing about PDQ is that it should allow physicians in every community to instantly have access to all the latest information, accurate and up-to-the-minute from major cancer centers worldwide. The net result should be the saving of pain, suffering, expense and many lives.

Q. How do I know I'm getting the right treatment for my cancer?

A. That is an excellent question. Cancer is a very serious disease. You generally have one chance to beat it. If you fail to treat it properly the first time, often there is no second chance.

Your question, however, shows much more than that. I believe it takes three things to beat cancer: a strong desire to live, complete faith in your doctor and confidence that the treatments that you are receiving will successfully treat you. Your question demonstrates that you lack the last two requisites.

I have two suggestions. You may want to call the Cancer Information Service at 1-800-4-CANCER. This is a toll-free service of the National Cancer Institute. Their purpose is to give you any factual information about your cancer that you care to know. The other suggestion is to get a second opinion from a qualified physician specializing in your type of cancer or, if possible, from a multidisciplinary panel.

Get the answers so that you can have full confidence in your physicians without any doubts. Then you have the best chance of beating this disease.

Q. What are the monoclonal antibodies that I have been reading a lot about?

A. A monoclonal antibody is a minute substance that will attach itself only to a particular type of cell for the purpose of delivering a treatment directly to that cell or being able to mark that cell.

Often, monoclonal antibodies are armed with a radioactive substance. They will go directly to a cancer cell, attach themselves and destroy this cell. Those that do not locate a cancer cell promptly lose their potency and become innocuous. Monoclonal antibodies are currently available for more than 20 types of cancer.

At a National Cancer Advisory Board meeting, we were told of a new monoclonal antibody to aid as a marker for ovarian cancer. Formerly, a woman with ovarian cancer had surgery followed by a year of chemotherapy. The only way to make certain she was cancer-free was to have a "second-look" surgery. Now, a small quantity of blood taken from her can be treated with a monoclonal antibody to show with 80 percent accuracy whether she is free of cancer. During the year of chemotherapy, her blood tests can be used to show whether she is improving or regressing. The actual cost of the test is approximately $130. The progress of modern medicine is rapid and mind-boggling.

Q. I would like to get a second opinion about treating my cancer. My doctor has been our family physician for years, and I don't want to hurt his feelings.

A. An outstanding oncologist once told me he has never treated a cancer patient without a second opinion, for four reasons. First, cancer is a very serious disease and, if you do not treat it properly the first time, generally there is no second chance. Second, somebody else could see something that he does not see. Third, somebody else could have some knowledge that he does not have. Fourth, he is a human being and he could make a mistake.

After hearing this, I came to the conclusion that any doctor treating cancer without a second opinion is not practicing medicine but trying to play God, because supposedly it is only God who is perfect, sees everything, knows everything and never makes a mistake.

The critical thing is to find a qualified physician in whom you have confidence who says he can successfully treat you.

The physician should be an oncologist, which is a doctor trained to specifically treat cancer. You must have confidence in your physician and be able to communicate well with him. This will enable you to understand and be involved with your treatment.

Finally, if your doctor says you will not make it, you have absolutely nothing to lose by trying to find a qualified doctor who believes he can successfully treat you or an institution that is doing successful research.

This is your life, and you must think of yourself first. I have never met a good doctor yet who did not welcome a second opinion. It can only reinforce your confidence in him and enable you to be more receptive to your treatment.

Q. My doctor wants me to take chemotherapy after surgery and radiation for my breast cancer. A friend of mine was cured with only a lumpectomy and radiation. Why should I have to take chemotherapy?

A. No two cases of cancer are identical. Each case is as unique as a fingerprint. Don't ever compare yourself to anyone else. Your cancer is one of at least 100 different types, one of numerous cell types further differentiated to a specific degree. Upon discovery, it was at a specific stage, had grown to a certain size and had or had not metastasized to other areas of your body. Your general physical condition, along with your age and mental attitude, are yours alone. The support from your family and friends and your faith in God is unique and applies only to you.

Don't compare yourself to anyone else and certainly don't compare yourself to a statistic.

If you have any questions about what your doctor recommends, ask your doctor. Explain why you are asking and what your concerns are. He will be happy to point out the differences and show why he is recommending what he is.

Q. I read that the government is spending more than $1 billion a year for cancer research. I also read that more than 555,500 Americans will die from cancer this year. Is the money we are spending wasted?

A. Dr. Charles LeMaistre, past president of M.D. Anderson in Houston, one of America's leading cancer centers, was quoted as saying, "And now for the first time we see more than 62 percent of all cancer patients being cured, making cancer the most curable of all chronic illnesses."

When I was appointed to the National Cancer Advisory Board, Dr. Vincent T. DeVita, Jr., former director of the National Cancer Institute, told us that progress was being made so rapidly that research projects started six months before were already obsolete. The next year, he told us that any physician who had not studied the current treatment for a specific cancer since yesterday could be out of date today. Furthermore, many of the cancers a physician graduating from medical school 20 years ago was taught were incurable are today curable to some degree.

In my opinion, the American public is getting a least $1.25 value for every $1 spent.

Q. A friend suggested I stop my present treatments, as they are making me very weak and sick. She showed me an article about people who are being cured by going out of the country to such places as Mexico, the

Bahamas, Greece and Germany for alternative therapies. What are your feelings?

A. First of all, let's be very clear what is meant by alternative therapies. These are methods of treating cancer that have not been scientifically proven and are always given in place of legitimate, orthodox medical treatments.

There is no magic bullet. There is no easy way out. Nothing can replace sound, tried and proven medical treatments.

It is human nature to look for an easy solution and avoid unpleasant treatments. It is my personal feeling that some individuals are driven to alternative therapies because all hope has been taken away, and a human being will not be denied hope. We are not talking about supplemental therapies that are recommended in addition to medical treatment, not in lieu of. By supplemental therapies, I mean prayers, psychotherapy and certain diets and vitamins taken with the approval of your physician. Again, let me stress that these are only in addition to proper medical treatments and not instead of.

My suggestion is to totally ignore this bad advice and to continue to follow your doctor's recommendations. Be grateful that your treatments have been discovered and perfected and that your doctor is so knowledgeable and caring. Remember, if these treatments are making you so tired and sick, think of what they are doing to those weak, little cancer cells.

Q. I read about your mental attitude quiz. Has it proved valid?

A. In the instructions, it states, "This test is not scientifically proven accurate." When this test was compiled, it was reviewed, and advice and suggestions were incorporated from psychiatrists, psychologists and physicians at Memorial Sloan-Kettering, the National Cancer Institute and in Kansas City. This quiz encompasses the various factors to indicate whether a patient does or does not have the proper mental attitude to be successfully treated for cancer in the opinion of these experts.

Even more important than that, this quiz presents the possibility of helping many cancer patients without any downside risks. There is no chance of hurting anyone. It is not intended to change anyone's ideas. It will either indicate that a positive person has the right mental outlook or that an individual should seek competent assistance. It is meant to aid your physician and augment your medical treatment. Remember that, in fighting cancer, you muster all your resources and do everything possible to try to beat this disease.

The feedback we have received from those who have taken the quiz shows that it has been a positive and helpful step for many. It is on page 114. Additional copies can be obtained, absolutely free of charge, by sending a stamped, self-addressed envelope to: R.A. Bloch Cancer Foundation, 4400 Main St., Kansas City, MO 64111.

Q. I'm so angry at myself that I didn't stop smoking sooner. I keep asking myself if I could have avoided getting cancer if I had quit a few years ago.

A. What's the difference? Why torture yourself? The important thing now is to cure your cancer. A vital ingredient is to never look back and have guilt feelings.

Every individual has a limited amount of energy. Don't waste precious energy looking back. You must muster all your resources and apply them toward your recovery. Turn these negative questions and doubts into positive thoughts of cooperation with your physician. In the two years of my treatments, not a single doctor asked me if I had been a smoker. It was perfectly obvious that I had, but what good would it have done to make me feel guilty?

You have lots of options that require all your energies in addition to receiving the treatments recommended by your physician. They include support from your family and friends; faith in God; being certain you receive proper, well-balanced nutrition; reading and learning more about your condition and treatment; and maintaining a positive mental attitude.

Q. Why do you feel that I should have detailed knowledge of my cancer and my treatments? I have full confidence in my physician and I would rather be spared the gory details.

A. An outstanding radiation oncologist in Detroit explains in detail to new patients all the factors about their cancer and the forthcoming treatments. When the oncologist is finished, he gives patients a tape recording of the entire interview to take home. He knows that if he had not given them the tape they would have worried about many things in the future that he had explained, but which they would have forgotten. He believes that the worry would be detrimental to their condition, while a thorough understanding would contribute to the success of the treatments.

The National Cancer Institute sent to the directors of 110 cancer centers the following poster, with the recommendation that it be placed in patient waiting areas over the director's signature.

Notice to patients: To obtain maximum benefit from your treatment, become a partner with your physician. You should understand everything being done for you and how and why it works. To do this you must ask questions! Your doctor wants you to understand, but will not know your concerns unless you express them. A physician or nurse will take as much time as necessary to explain anything about your condition that you do not understand. A partnership like this will ensure that the care you receive is optimal.

Q. My father was told he has terminal cancer with no treatments possible. He was told he has about two years to live. Is there nothing he can do?

A. First of all, I believe you should clearly define the meaning of the word "terminal." Supposedly, terminal means dying imminently from an existing condition from which there is no possibility of altering the outcome. My understanding of this would not include an individual who has as much as two years to live.

There are many documented cases of individuals who were told they were going to die from their cancer, with no possible treatment, only to be seen years later alive, well and cancer-free.

There is a phenomenon known as spontaneous remission that medical science has been unable to explain to date. It is where cancer completely disappears for no apparent reason.

With all the tremendous advances being made daily in cancer treatments, there is always hope. Who knows what will be discovered within the two years allotted for your father that will be applicable to him?

In my opinion, "terminal" means dying this afternoon or tomorrow or this week. I am not trying to say that your father can be successfully treated, but I would urge him to seek a second opinion. Staying with a doctor who says there is no hope will generally fulfill his prophecy.

Q. Why is your Cancer Hot Line different from all the other groups available.

A. There are many wonderful and helpful support groups available.

Primarily, the Cancer Hot Line is a group of individuals who have had cancer who are available to talk to newly diagnosed cancer patients, ideally within 15 minutes of their diagnosis.

We do not make a prognosis or give medical advice. We talk strictly from personal experience, emphasizing prompt treatment, proper treatment, thorough treatment and a positive mental attitude.

Psychologically, we enable them to get over the initial shock and fear and to understand that death and cancer are not synonymous. The patient realizes that, because they are talking to someone who has had a similar cancer, it is possible for them to overcome it. However, we give a lot more than psychological help.

We recommend the patient consult a qualified physician, such as an oncologist. Because we do not solicit cash contributions from any patient we are free to suggest any qualified physician we personally like. We further recommend a qualified second opinion, because we know how serious cancer is and no one is perfect.

We try to help them find a qualified doctor in whom they have faith who says he can successfully treat them. If this doctor cannot be found, we then try to get them to the institution that is doing the most successful work on their type of cancer.

Because we have been there with a similar cancer, we can explain in lay terms what the treatments their doctor recommends are like and how they affected us. We can give practical hints on what we did to help ourselves. We try to take fear of the unknown out of cancer treatment. We attempt to get the callers in control of their cancer and to become more of a partner with their doctor.

We recommend to each patient that they read *Fighting Cancer* and *CANCER...there's hope*, available free by requesting them from 1-800-433-0464, or through our website: www.blochcancer.org.

We believe we improve the quality of life for every patient and extend the quantity of life for many. Our sole goal is to give the next person getting cancer the best chance of beating it.

The Cancer Hot Line number is 1-800-433-0464.

Check List 14

Carefully read each statement and place a ✔ in ☐ where true.

☐ I am starting off with a positive mental attitude.

☐ I do not compare myself with anyone else.

☐ I do not think of why I got cancer.

☐ I do not think of why I did not discover my cancer earlier.

☐ I do not think of what caused my cancer.

☐ I really have a strong desire to get well.

☐ I am having my cancer treated as promptly as possible.

☐ I have a doctor who is qualified to treat cancer.

☐ I have a doctor who says he can successfully treat me.

☐ I have a doctor who is totally honest with me.

☐ I have a doctor who takes time to explain everything about my cancer.

☐ I have a doctor who answers all my questions so that I understand.

☐ I have a doctor who I can call anytime when something bothers me.

☐ I have a doctor who has my complete confidence.

☐ I have a doctor who is giving me a treatment I believe will be successful.

☐ I have gotten a qualified second opinion.

☐ I do not worry about hurting my doctor's feelings.

☐ I make lists of questions to ask my doctor.

☐ I am willing to do anything my doctor says I must.

☐ I take a friend or relative with me when I visit my doctor.

☐ I take a tape recorder when I visit my doctor.

☐ I make every effort to take each treatment on schedule.

☐ I have nothing that is important enough to postpone a cancer treatment for.

☐ I appreciate the sacrifices others made so I may take treatments.

☐ I am taking the pain medication the way the doctor recommends it.

☐ I am finding out all I can about my disease.

☐ I have called 1-800-4-CANCER to find the state-of-the-art therapy on PDQ.

☐ I eat a well-balanced diet.

☐ I make myself eat enough to maintain my weight.

☐ I do not smoke.

☐ I have a strong support group of family and/or friends.

☐ I let my support group know how much I appreciate and need them.

☐ I confide in my support group.

☐ I am happy to answer anyone's questions about how I feel.

☐ I am willing to discuss my problems with my family or friends.

☐ I ask my family or friends for help whenever I need it.

☐ I continuously state that I am going to do everything to beat this disease.

☐ I try to talk out anything that bothers me.

☐ I set aside time daily for my personal pleasure.

☐ I expose myself to humor and laugh whenever possible.

☐ I am being selfish in that I am doing what I believe is best for myself.

☐ I give in to myself and rest when I get tired.

☐ I lead a full life, trying to keep my activities as close to normal as possible.

☐ I exercise regularly.

☐ I have pleasant activities planned for whenever I may become depressed.

- [ ] I change my thoughts when I become depressed.

- [ ] I have goals to shoot for and projects to complete.

- [ ] I practice relaxation and imagery 3 times a day.

- [ ] I have taken the mental attitude quiz.

- [ ] I am finished with any emotional problems I may have had in the past.

- [ ] I believe the good things that have happened to me far outweigh the bad.

- [ ] I am not afraid to die.

- [ ] I say a prayer at least daily.

- [ ] I am confident that when cancer is behind me, it will never come back.

- [ ] I am making plans for things to do when I am well.

- [ ] I am keeping busy and doing everything I am capable of doing.

- [ ] I feel I am in charge.

- [ ] I have made a commitment and am doing everything I can to beat my cancer.

Stop! If you did not honestly check the list, go back and check the boxes that are true. This book was written for one purpose, the same reason you have read it — to help you fight cancer! Go back and re-read each statement that you did not check. Be positive! Start with the assumption that everything applies to you. Don't be negative. Don't assume anything may be fine for someone else but not for you. That particular constructive suggestion is particularly for you! Don't knock it until you have tried it. After you give it a fair trial, then and only then can you honestly say it isn't for you.

Fighting cancer is not a simple matter of thinking positively, wishing it away and saying "Hey, Doc, cure me." It is a matter of knowledge. It is a matter of educating yourself about every detail and mustering all your resources. Use every drop of energy in an organized fashion to constructively concentrate on getting rid of cancer. Most cancers can be successfully treated, but generally you have only one chance. If you miss that first chance, if you don't do everything in your power, often there is no second chance. This is why no cancer patient can afford the luxury of looking back and saying "I wish I would have..." Never look back. Concentrate on this moment forward and do everything in your power. There is no downside risk. Now you may have a chance. Good luck and God bless you.

Thx Importancx of Propxr Trxatmxnt

Xvxn though my typxwritxr is an old modxl, it works rathxr wxll xxcxpt for onx of thx kxys. I'vx wishxd many timxs that it workxd propxrly. It's trux that thxrx arx forty-six othxr kxys that function wxll xnough, but just onx kxy not working makxs thx dif-fxrxncx.

Cancxr trxatmxnt is likx my typxwritxr. Xvxry phasx of it must bx propxr for it to havx a chancx of coming out right. If you arx unfor-tunatx xnough to bx thx onx in thrxx who gxts cancxr, if you go through all thx mxntal pain and suffxring along with your family and frixnds, if you takx all thx trxatmxnts and do all thx things you should xxcxpt for maybx onx, your rxsults may comx out just likx this pagx.

But there is a big difference! Your life probably·cannot be erased and corrected after it has been improperly treated like this sheet of paper, even if forty-six out of forty-seven things have been done correctly.

About the Authors

Richard A. (Dick) Bloch, born in Kansas City, Missouri on February 15, 1926, is the youngest of three sons. An entrepreneur at heart, at age nine he bought a hand printing press and started a business. He was so successful that by his twelfth birthday he had progressed to three automatic presses and was doing much of the printing for all the high schools in Kansas City. After high school, he sold his business to a college in Iowa as a model shop for use in printing courses.

Dick attended the Wharton School of Finance at the University of Pennsylvania where he received a bachelor of science degree in economics at the age of 19. While in college, he bought cars, took them apart, put them back together and then sold them to pay for his expenses. After graduation, Bloch joined his older brother, Henry, in the formation of a bookkeeping and tax preparation company. They started a new company in 1955 specializing in tax preparation, H&R Block, Inc. The world's largest tax services company, H&R Block in fiscal year 2002 served nearly 23 million tax clients in approximately 10,400 retail offices worldwide.

In 1978, Dick was told he had terminal lung cancer with 3 months to live. Refusing to accept this prognosis, he went to a major comprehensive cancer center where, after 2 years of aggressive therapy, he was told he was cured. Since Bloch's bout with cancer, he has focused his attention on working "to help the next person who gets cancer." He sold his interest in H&R Block, Inc. and retired from the company in 1982 to be able to devote all his efforts to cancer.

Richard and Annette Bloch are founders of the Cancer Hot Line in Kansas City, a volunteer organization of more than 500 cancer patients which has received more than 200,000 calls from newly diagnosed cancer patients since its inception in 1980.

On September 2, 1980, the Cancer Treatment Panel started meeting weekly in various hospitals seeing 3 or 4 patients to offer a multidisciplinary second opinion. This was changed to the R. A. Bloch Cancer Management Center at the University of Missouri-Kansas City on May 1, 1982 meeting twice a week. Newly diagnosed patients appeared in front of a medical, surgical and radiation oncologist, diagnostic radiologist, pathologist and psychologist to hear each discuss their particular case and receive recommendations. There was no charge to the patient, and the doctors volunteered their time. This operated so successfully that all the patients who wanted to come could not be accommodated. Eighteen institutions geographically distributed around the U.S. were recruited to assist and offered the same service. By 1995, demand caused the service to be discontinued in favor of 6 hospitals in the Kansas City area offering it. The goal is to enroll some 1,500 institutions nationally. Currently, well over 100 institutions nationally are offering multidisciplinary second opinions.

From May 1, 1988 to October 2001, the R. A. Bloch Cancer Support Center served cancer patients on the grounds of the University of Missouri - Kansas City. It was a relaxing, comfortable place for patients and their supporters to congregate for the purposes of sharing and education. This was coordinated by professionals and like all other Bloch programs, was completely free.

Dick developed a computer program which the National Cancer Institute has implemented under the name "PDQ" for "Physicians Data Query." It gives the state-of-the-art treatment for every type and stage of cancer and all the current open experimental therapies. This information is gathered from every cancer center in the United States and over 100 foreign countries and is continuously updated by a staff of 72 researchers. In government publications it states, "If physicians avail themselves of the opportunity now offered by PDQ, the NCI estimates the national survival rates would rise by at least 10% or more than 50,000 lives per year." The government named the building housing this program in Bethesda, MD, the R.A. Bloch International

Cancer Information Center. Most government issued cancer information emanates from this building.

Dick & Annette are the authors of 3 books. *Cancer...there's hope* is a story of Richard and Annette's fight against his "terminal" lung cancer. It is written, not to tell a story, but to show others what they can do to battle this disease. *Fighting Cancer* is a step-by-step guide for cancer patients to help themselves fight the disease. These 2 books are both available free in public libraries or by calling the Cancer Hotline at 1-800-433-0464, or through www.blochcancer.org. Their latest book, *Guide for Cancer Supporters* is written to help supporters exclusively. It is available free by calling the Cancer Hot Line at 1- 800-433-0464.

They started the Fighting Cancer Rally in 1986 to demonstrate that death and cancer are not synonymous and that there is a possibility of a quality of life after the diagnosis of cancer. Over 700 rallies now are held, simultaneously, across the country the first Sunday in June. At the rally in Kansas City in June, 1990, the first

R.A. Bloch Cancer Survivor's park was dedicated to the 5,000,000 living Americans who had been diagnosed with cancer, 2,000,000 of whom were considered cured. Today those figures have nearly doubled! Other parks are completed or nearing completion in Bakersfield, Baltimore, Chicago, Cleveland, Columbus, Dallas, Houston, Indianapolis, Jacksonville, Minneapolis, New Orleans, Omaha, Phoenix, Rancho Mirage, Sacramento, San Diego, Santa Rosa, Tampa, and Tucson.

Annette and Dick talk to over 1,000 cancer patients individually each year, listening to their problems and trying to help them and their families. They go around the country speaking to different groups and organizations. They have been the subject of articles in numerous magazines including *Family Circle*, *Medical World News*, *People*, *Cosmopolitan*, *Vogue*, *Forbes*, and *Reader's Digest*. They have appeared on national television on every major network and in numerous documentaries. They have received awards or been honored by such organizations as the American Cancer Society, the Sertoma Club, the Department of Health and Human Services, the Rotary Club, the Lion's Club, Church of Jesus Christ of Latter-day Saints, and they received the Mankind Award from Cystic Fibrosis. In 1982, Dick was appointed by President Reagan to the National Cancer Advisory Board for a 6 year term. In 1989, he was selected as one of the "Most caring individuals" from 4,000 nominees by the Caring Institute in Washington. He is a member of the President's Circle of the National Academy of Sciences, the Institute of Medicine and was on the NIH's Office of Alternative Medicine for 2 years. Dick received the American Society of Clinical Oncology's Public Service Award in 1994 "in recognition of exemplary contributions to the field of oncology and to patients with cancer." He received the 1995 Layman's Award from the Society of Surgical Oncology at their Annual Convention.

Annette Modell Bloch was born in Philadelphia, Pennsylvania, where she lived until her marriage to Dick in 1946. She and Dick have three daughters - Barbara, Nancy and Linda and ten grandchildren. Her family always her top priority, Annette has also participated in many civic activities and is now Dick's partner in all of their cancer projects including public appearances and talks to various groups. Annette and Dick received *Coping* magazine's 1995 Hero Award for Lifetime Achievement.

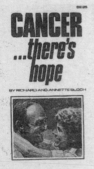

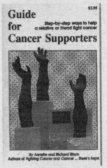

Explaining in lay
terms what cancer
is and what a
patient can do to
help himself.

Step-by-Step ways
to help a relative or
friend fight cancer.

**Available free
by calling
1-800-433-0464
or on our website www.blochcancer.org.**

If your library does not have *Cancer...there's hope*
or *Guide for Cancer Supporters*, they may get 2
copies free postpaid by sending a request on their
stationery to Cancer Hot Line, 4400 Main St.,
Kansas City, MO 64111.

The first book is free to any cancer patient by calling 1-800-433-0464. If you would like to order more copies, please complete the following order form.

Fighting Cancer is $4.*
Cancer...there's hope is $3*
Guide for Cancer Supporters is $3*
*Prices include postage.

Please send me:
_____ copies of *Fighting Cancer*
_____ copies of *Cancer...there's hope*
_____ copies of *Guide for Cancer Supporters*

I enclose $ _____*. This money will be used for cancer projects.

Mr./Mrs./Ms. _____

Address _____

City _____

State _____ Zip _____

Mail to: Cancer Hot Line
            4400 Main Street
            Kansas City, MO 64111